My Information

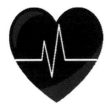

Name ....
Phone ....
Email ....
Address ....
....
Blood Type ....

Medical Contacts

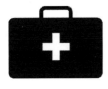

Doctor ....
Dentist ....
Specialist ....
Pharmacist ....

ICE Contact (CONTACT IN EMERGENCY)

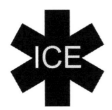

Name ....
Phone ....
Address ....
....

MEDICAL DISCLAIMER

Information in this book **IS NOT** intended to serve as a substitute for diagnosis, treatment, or advice from a qualified, licensed medical professional.

Any health guidelines you decide to follow should be discussed with your doctor or other licensed medical professional should you be unsure regarding your own specific health requirements.

If you have any health concerns or worries seek medical attention as soon as possible.

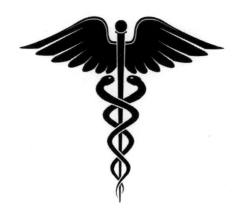

Copyright © 2020 Narooma Online Designs - All Rights Reserved

No part of this publication may be reproduced, stored in a retrieval system, or transmitted in any form or by any means, electronic, mechanical, photocopying, recording or otherwise, without the prior written permission of the publisher.

HOW TO USE THIS FOOD DIARY & TRACKER

The Low FODMAP Food Diary & IBS Tracker has been specifically designed to help you monitor your daily intake of food and drinks plus help you identify which foods do or don't suit you. It is clearly and simply laid out making it a simple job to complete each day.

Identifying which foods are causing your Irritable Bowel Syndrome can be frustrating when you can't target the culprit, especially since food reactions vary from person to person. We developed this specially tailored IBS Diary so that YOU could pinpoint your trigger foods simply and easily.

The Low FODMAP Food Diary and IBS Tracker has been divided into 3 main sections to simplify gathering and organizing your information:

1 Physical Trackers
2 Appointments & Records
3 Low FODMAP Foods, Meal Planners & Shopping Lists

By using this IBS Diary on a daily basis, you can develop a complete and accurate record of all aspects of your diet and any symptomatic reactions that occur enabling you to move forward with your meal planning.

Maintaining these trackers and diary regularly will provide you with a unique perspective of your health, assist you in identifying problem foods that cause negative reactions and will help you to manage your eating and avoid digestive and IBS issues in the future.

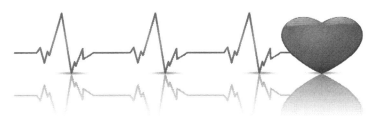

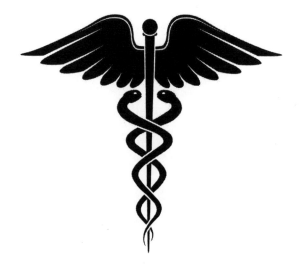

SECTION 1

PHYSICAL TRACKERS

Daily IBS Diary

Date: 31.7.20

BREAKFAST TIME:

FOOD & DRINK
1) Muesli
   with milk

INTENSITY/REACTION
LOW 01 ✓ 02 03
04 05 06
07 ✗ 08 09
10 11 12 HIGH

LUNCH TIME:

FOOD & DRINK
Cheese Strip
+ 2 chocolate biscuits

INTENSITY/REACTION
LOW 01 02 03
04 05 06
07 08 09
10 11 12 HIGH

DINNER TIME:

FOOD & DRINK
Glass wine
Campbell's cream
soup, yoghurt
biscuit

INTENSITY/REACTION
LOW 01 02 03
04 05 06
07 08 09
10 11 12 HIGH

SYMPTOMS -

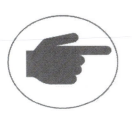

PAIN MEASUREMENT SCALE

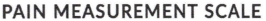
0 1 2 3 4 5 6 7 8 9 10

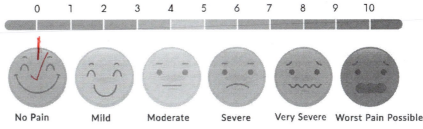
No Pain ✓ — Mild — Moderate — Severe — Very Severe — Worst Pain Possible

WATER TRACKER
1 2 3 4
5 6 7 8

STRESS LEVEL
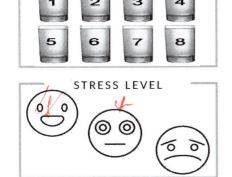

BRISTOL STOOL CHART

TYPE 1 – HARD LUMPS ☐
TYPE 2 – LUMPY ☐
TYPE 3 – CRACKED ☐
TYPE 4 – SMOOTH ☐
TYPE 5 – SOFT BLOBS ✓
TYPE 6 – MUSHY EDGES ☐
TYPE 7 – JUST LIQUID ☐

NOTES

Daily IBS Diary

Date: ....

BREAKFAST TIME: _____

FOOD & DRINK

Meusli
Melon
coffee

INTENSITY/REACTION

LOW → 01, 02, 03, 04, 05, 06, 07, 08, 09, 10, 11, 12 HIGH

LUNCH TIME: _____

FOOD & DRINK

quiche
salad
1 wine
granola

INTENSITY/REACTION

LOW → 01, 02, 03, 04, 05, 06, 07, 08, 09, 10, 11, 12 HIGH

DINNER TIME: _____

FOOD & DRINK

1 egg
bread
2 biscuits

INTENSITY/REACTION

LOW → 01, 02, 03, 04, 05, 06, 07, 08, 09, 10, 11, 12 HIGH

SYMPTOMS -

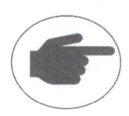

PAIN MEASUREMENT SCALE

0 1 2 3 4 5 6 7 8 9 10

No Pain | Mild | Moderate | Severe | Very Severe | Worst Pain Possible

WATER TRACKER

1 ✓ 2 3 4
5 6 7 8

STRESS LEVEL

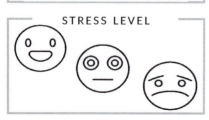

BRISTOL STOOL CHART

TYPE 1 – HARD LUMPS ☐
TYPE 2 – LUMPY ☐
TYPE 3 – CRACKED ☐
TYPE 4 – SMOOTH ☐
TYPE 5 – SOFT BLOBS ✓
TYPE 6 – MUSHY EDGES ☐
TYPE 7 – JUST LIQUID ☐

NOTES

Daily IBS Diary

Date: ....

BREAKFAST TIME: _____

FOOD & DRINK

INTENSITY/REACTION

LOW
01 02 03
04 05 06
07 08 09
10 11 12
HIGH

LUNCH TIME: _____

FOOD & DRINK

INTENSITY/REACTION

LOW
01 02 03
04 05 06
07 08 09
10 11 12
HIGH

DINNER TIME: _____

FOOD & DRINK

INTENSITY/REACTION

LOW
01 02 03
04 05 06
07 08 09
10 11 12
HIGH

SYMPTOMS -

PAIN MEASUREMENT SCALE

0 1 2 3 4 5 6 7 8 9 10

No Pain | Mild | Moderate | Severe | Very Severe | Worst Pain Possible

WATER TRACKER

1 2 3 4
5 6 7 8

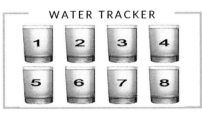

STRESS LEVEL

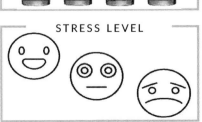

BRISTOL STOOL CHART

TYPE 1 – HARD LUMPS ☐

TYPE 2 – LUMPY ☐

TYPE 3 – CRACKED ☐

TYPE 4 – SMOOTH ☐

TYPE 5 – SOFT BLOBS ☐

TYPE 6 – MUSHY EDGES ☐

TYPE 7 – JUST LIQUID ☐

NOTES

Daily IBS Diary

Date: ....

BREAKFAST TIME: _____

FOOD & DRINK

INTENSITY/REACTION

LOW
- 01
- 02
- 03
- 04
- 05
- 06
- 07
- 08
- 09
- 10
- 11
- 12
HIGH

LUNCH TIME: _____

FOOD & DRINK

INTENSITY/REACTION

LOW
- 01
- 02
- 03
- 04
- 05
- 06
- 07
- 08
- 09
- 10
- 11
- 12
HIGH

DINNER TIME: _____

FOOD & DRINK

INTENSITY/REACTION

LOW
- 01
- 02
- 03
- 04
- 05
- 06
- 07
- 08
- 09
- 10
- 11
- 12
HIGH

SYMPTOMS -

PAIN MEASUREMENT SCALE

0 1 2 3 4 5 6 7 8 9 10

No Pain | Mild | Moderate | Severe | Very Severe | Worst Pain Possible

WATER TRACKER

1 2 3 4
5 6 7 8

STRESS LEVEL

BRISTOL STOOL CHART

TYPE 1 – HARD LUMPS ☐

TYPE 2 – LUMPY ☐

TYPE 3 – CRACKED ☐

TYPE 4 – SMOOTH ☐

TYPE 5 – SOFT BLOBS ☐

TYPE 6 – MUSHY EDGES ☐

TYPE 7 – JUST LIQUID ☐

NOTES

Daily IBS Diary

Date: ....

BREAKFAST TIME: _____

FOOD & DRINK

INTENSITY/REACTION

LOW
01 02 03
04 05 06
07 08 09
10 11 12
HIGH

LUNCH TIME: _____

FOOD & DRINK

INTENSITY/REACTION

LOW
01 02 03
04 05 06
07 08 09
10 11 12
HIGH

DINNER TIME: _____

FOOD & DRINK

INTENSITY/REACTION

LOW
01 02 03
04 05 06
07 08 09
10 11 12
HIGH

SYMPTOMS -

PAIN MEASUREMENT SCALE

0 1 2 3 4 5 6 7 8 9 10

No Pain | Mild | Moderate | Severe | Very Severe | Worst Pain Possible

WATER TRACKER
1 2 3 4
5 6 7 8

STRESS LEVEL

BRISTOL STOOL CHART

TYPE 1 – HARD LUMPS ☐

TYPE 2 – LUMPY ☐

TYPE 3 – CRACKED ☐

TYPE 4 – SMOOTH ☐

TYPE 5 – SOFT BLOBS ☐

TYPE 6 – MUSHY EDGES ☐

TYPE 7 – JUST LIQUID ☐

NOTES

Daily IBS Diary

Date: ....

BREAKFAST TIME: _____

FOOD & DRINK

INTENSITY/REACTION

LOW 01 02 03
04 05 06
07 08 09
10 11 12 HIGH

LUNCH TIME: _____

FOOD & DRINK

INTENSITY/REACTION

LOW 01 02 03
04 05 06
07 08 09
10 11 12 HIGH

DINNER TIME: _____

FOOD & DRINK

INTENSITY/REACTION

LOW 01 02 03
04 05 06
07 08 09
10 11 12 HIGH

SYMPTOMS -

PAIN MEASUREMENT SCALE

0 1 2 3 4 5 6 7 8 9 10

No Pain | Mild | Moderate | Severe | Very Severe | Worst Pain Possible

WATER TRACKER

1 2 3 4
5 6 7 8

STRESS LEVEL

BRISTOL STOOL CHART

TYPE 1 – HARD LUMPS ☐

TYPE 2 – LUMPY ☐

TYPE 3 – CRACKED ☐

TYPE 4 – SMOOTH ☐

TYPE 5 – SOFT BLOBS ☐

TYPE 6 – MUSHY EDGES ☐

TYPE 7 – JUST LIQUID ☐

NOTES

Daily IBS Diary

Date: ....

BREAKFAST TIME: _____

FOOD & DRINK

INTENSITY/REACTION

LOW
01 02 03
04 05 06
07 08 09
10 11 12
HIGH

LUNCH TIME: _____

FOOD & DRINK

INTENSITY/REACTION

LOW
01 02 03
04 05 06
07 08 09
10 11 12
HIGH

DINNER TIME: _____

FOOD & DRINK

INTENSITY/REACTION

LOW
01 02 03
04 05 06
07 08 09
10 11 12
HIGH

SYMPTOMS -

PAIN MEASUREMENT SCALE

0 1 2 3 4 5 6 7 8 9 10

No Pain | Mild | Moderate | Severe | Very Severe | Worst Pain Possible

WATER TRACKER

1 2 3 4
5 6 7 8

STRESS LEVEL

BRISTOL STOOL CHART

TYPE 1 – HARD LUMPS ☐

TYPE 2 – LUMPY ☐

TYPE 3 – CRACKED ☐

TYPE 4 – SMOOTH ☐

TYPE 5 – SOFT BLOBS ☐

TYPE 6 – MUSHY EDGES ☐

TYPE 7 – JUST LIQUID ☐

NOTES

Daily IBS Diary

Date: ....

BREAKFAST TIME: _____

FOOD & DRINK

INTENSITY/REACTION

LOW 01 02 03
04 05 06
07 08 09
10 11 12 HIGH

LUNCH TIME: _____

FOOD & DRINK

INTENSITY/REACTION

LOW 01 02 03
04 05 06
07 08 09
10 11 12 HIGH

DINNER TIME: _____

FOOD & DRINK

INTENSITY/REACTION

LOW 01 02 03
04 05 06
07 08 09
10 11 12 HIGH

SYMPTOMS -

PAIN MEASUREMENT SCALE

0 1 2 3 4 5 6 7 8 9 10

No Pain | Mild | Moderate | Severe | Very Severe | Worst Pain Possible

WATER TRACKER

1 2 3 4
5 6 7 8

STRESS LEVEL

BRISTOL STOOL CHART

TYPE 1 – HARD LUMPS ☐
TYPE 2 – LUMPY ☐
TYPE 3 – CRACKED ☐
TYPE 4 – SMOOTH ☐
TYPE 5 – SOFT BLOBS ☐
TYPE 6 – MUSHY EDGES ☐
TYPE 7 – JUST LIQUID ☐

NOTES

Daily IBS Diary

Date: ....

BREAKFAST TIME: _____

LUNCH TIME: _____

DINNER TIME: _____

FOOD & DRINK

INTENSITY/REACTION

LOW
01 02 03
04 05 06
07 08 09
10 11 12
HIGH

FOOD & DRINK

INTENSITY/REACTION

LOW
01 02 03
04 05 06
07 08 09
10 11 12
HIGH

FOOD & DRINK

INTENSITY/REACTION

LOW
01 02 03
04 05 06
07 08 09
10 11 12
HIGH

SYMPTOMS -

PAIN MEASUREMENT SCALE

0 1 2 3 4 5 6 7 8 9 10

No Pain | Mild | Moderate | Severe | Very Severe | Worst Pain Possible

WATER TRACKER

1 2 3 4
5 6 7 8

STRESS LEVEL

BRISTOL STOOL CHART

TYPE 1 – HARD LUMPS ☐

TYPE 2 – LUMPY ☐

TYPE 3 – CRACKED ☐

TYPE 4 – SMOOTH ☐

TYPE 5 – SOFT BLOBS ☐

TYPE 6 – MUSHY EDGES ☐

TYPE 7 – JUST LIQUID ☐

NOTES

Daily IBS Diary

Date: ....

BREAKFAST TIME: _____

LUNCH TIME: _____

DINNER TIME: _____

FOOD & DRINK

INTENSITY/REACTION

LOW
- 01 02 03
- 04 05 06
- 07 08 09
- 10 11 12
HIGH

FOOD & DRINK

INTENSITY/REACTION

LOW
- 01 02 03
- 04 05 06
- 07 08 09
- 10 11 12
HIGH

FOOD & DRINK

INTENSITY/REACTION

LOW
- 01 02 03
- 04 05 06
- 07 08 09
- 10 11 12
HIGH

SYMPTOMS -

PAIN MEASUREMENT SCALE

0 1 2 3 4 5 6 7 8 9 10

No Pain | Mild | Moderate | Severe | Very Severe | Worst Pain Possible

WATER TRACKER
1 2 3 4
5 6 7 8

STRESS LEVEL

BRISTOL STOOL CHART

TYPE 1 – HARD LUMPS ☐

TYPE 2 – LUMPY ☐

TYPE 3 – CRACKED ☐

TYPE 4 – SMOOTH ☐

TYPE 5 – SOFT BLOBS ☐

TYPE 6 – MUSHY EDGES ☐

TYPE 7 – JUST LIQUID ☐

NOTES

Daily IBS Diary

Date: ....

BREAKFAST TIME: _____

FOOD & DRINK

INTENSITY/REACTION

LOW 01 02 03
04 05 06
07 08 09
10 11 12 HIGH

LUNCH TIME: _____

FOOD & DRINK

INTENSITY/REACTION

LOW 01 02 03
04 05 06
07 08 09
10 11 12 HIGH

DINNER TIME: _____

FOOD & DRINK

INTENSITY/REACTION

LOW 01 02 03
04 05 06
07 08 09
10 11 12 HIGH

SYMPTOMS -

PAIN MEASUREMENT SCALE

0 1 2 3 4 5 6 7 8 9 10

No Pain | Mild | Moderate | Severe | Very Severe | Worst Pain Possible

WATER TRACKER

1 2 3 4
5 6 7 8

STRESS LEVEL

BRISTOL STOOL CHART

TYPE 1 – HARD LUMPS ☐

TYPE 2 – LUMPY ☐

TYPE 3 – CRACKED ☐

TYPE 4 – SMOOTH ☐

TYPE 5 – SOFT BLOBS ☐

TYPE 6 – MUSHY EDGES ☐

TYPE 7 – JUST LIQUID ☐

NOTES

Daily IBS Diary

Date: ....

BREAKFAST TIME: _____

FOOD & DRINK

INTENSITY/REACTION

LOW
- 01 02 03
- 04 05 06
- 07 08 09
- 10 11 12 HIGH

LUNCH TIME: _____

FOOD & DRINK

INTENSITY/REACTION

LOW
- 01 02 03
- 04 05 06
- 07 08 09
- 10 11 12 HIGH

DINNER TIME: _____

FOOD & DRINK

INTENSITY/REACTION

LOW
- 01 02 03
- 04 05 06
- 07 08 09
- 10 11 12 HIGH

SYMPTOMS -

PAIN MEASUREMENT SCALE

0 1 2 3 4 5 6 7 8 9 10

No Pain | Mild | Moderate | Severe | Very Severe | Worst Pain Possible

WATER TRACKER

1 2 3 4
5 6 7 8

STRESS LEVEL

BRISTOL STOOL CHART

TYPE 1 – HARD LUMPS ☐

TYPE 2 – LUMPY ☐

TYPE 3 – CRACKED ☐

TYPE 4 – SMOOTH ☐

TYPE 5 – SOFT BLOBS ☐

TYPE 6 – MUSHY EDGES ☐

TYPE 7 – JUST LIQUID ☐

NOTES

Daily IBS Diary

Date: ....

BREAKFAST TIME: _____

FOOD & DRINK

INTENSITY/REACTION

LOW
< 01 < 02 < 03
< 04 < 05 < 06
< 07 < 08 < 09
< 10 < 11 < 12
HIGH

LUNCH TIME: _____

FOOD & DRINK

INTENSITY/REACTION

LOW
< 01 < 02 < 03
< 04 < 05 < 06
< 07 < 08 < 09
< 10 < 11 < 12
HIGH

DINNER TIME: _____

FOOD & DRINK

INTENSITY/REACTION

LOW
< 01 < 02 < 03
< 04 < 05 < 06
< 07 < 08 < 09
< 10 < 11 < 12
HIGH

SYMPTOMS -

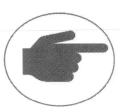

PAIN MEASUREMENT SCALE

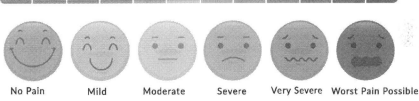

0 1 2 3 4 5 6 7 8 9 10

No Pain — Mild — Moderate — Severe — Very Severe — Worst Pain Possible

BRISTOL STOOL CHART

TYPE 1 – HARD LUMPS ☐

TYPE 2 – LUMPY ☐

TYPE 3 – CRACKED ☐

TYPE 4 – SMOOTH ☐

TYPE 5 – SOFT BLOBS ☐

TYPE 6 – MUSHY EDGES ☐

TYPE 7 – JUST LIQUID ☐

WATER TRACKER

1 2 3 4
5 6 7 8

STRESS LEVEL

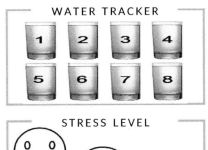

NOTES

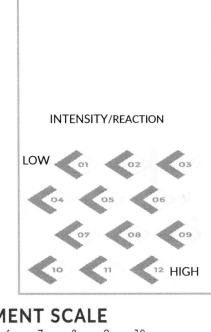

Daily IBS Diary

Date: ....

BREAKFAST TIME: _____

LUNCH TIME: _____

DINNER TIME: _____

FOOD & DRINK

INTENSITY/REACTION

LOW 01 02 03
04 05 06
07 08 09
10 11 12 HIGH

(Breakfast, Lunch, Dinner columns)

SYMPTOMS -

PAIN MEASUREMENT SCALE

0 1 2 3 4 5 6 7 8 9 10

No Pain — Mild — Moderate — Severe — Very Severe — Worst Pain Possible

WATER TRACKER
1 2 3 4
5 6 7 8

STRESS LEVEL

BRISTOL STOOL CHART

TYPE 1 – HARD LUMPS ☐
TYPE 2 – LUMPY ☐
TYPE 3 – CRACKED ☐
TYPE 4 – SMOOTH ☐
TYPE 5 – SOFT BLOBS ☐
TYPE 6 – MUSHY EDGES ☐
TYPE 7 – JUST LIQUID ☐

NOTES

Daily IBS Diary

Date: ....

BREAKFAST TIME: _____

FOOD & DRINK

INTENSITY/REACTION

LOW
< 01 < 02 < 03
< 04 < 05 < 06
< 07 < 08 < 09
< 10 < 11 < 12   HIGH

LUNCH TIME: _____

FOOD & DRINK

INTENSITY/REACTION

LOW
< 01 < 02 < 03
< 04 < 05 < 06
< 07 < 08 < 09
< 10 < 11 < 12   HIGH

DINNER TIME: _____

FOOD & DRINK

INTENSITY/REACTION

LOW
< 01 < 02 < 03
< 04 < 05 < 06
< 07 < 08 < 09
< 10 < 11 < 12   HIGH

SYMPTOMS -

PAIN MEASUREMENT SCALE

0 1 2 3 4 5 6 7 8 9 10

| No Pain | Mild | Moderate | Severe | Very Severe | Worst Pain Possible |

WATER TRACKER

1 2 3 4
5 6 7 8

STRESS LEVEL

BRISTOL STOOL CHART

TYPE 1 – HARD LUMPS ☐

TYPE 2 – LUMPY ☐

TYPE 3 – CRACKED ☐

TYPE 4 – SMOOTH ☐

TYPE 5 – SOFT BLOBS ☐

TYPE 6 – MUSHY EDGES ☐

TYPE 7 – JUST LIQUID ☐

NOTES

Daily IBS Diary

Date: ....

BREAKFAST TIME: _____

FOOD & DRINK

INTENSITY/REACTION

LOW
01 02 03
04 05 06
07 08 09
10 11 12 HIGH

LUNCH TIME: _____

FOOD & DRINK

INTENSITY/REACTION

LOW
01 02 03
04 05 06
07 08 09
10 11 12 HIGH

DINNER TIME: _____

FOOD & DRINK

INTENSITY/REACTION

LOW
01 02 03
04 05 06
07 08 09
10 11 12 HIGH

SYMPTOMS -

PAIN MEASUREMENT SCALE

0 1 2 3 4 5 6 7 8 9 10

No Pain | Mild | Moderate | Severe | Very Severe | Worst Pain Possible

WATER TRACKER
1 2 3 4
5 6 7 8

STRESS LEVEL

BRISTOL STOOL CHART

TYPE 1 – HARD LUMPS ☐
TYPE 2 – LUMPY ☐
TYPE 3 – CRACKED ☐
TYPE 4 – SMOOTH ☐
TYPE 5 – SOFT BLOBS ☐
TYPE 6 – MUSHY EDGES ☐
TYPE 7 – JUST LIQUID ☐

NOTES

Daily IBS Diary

Date: ....

BREAKFAST TIME: _____

FOOD & DRINK

INTENSITY/REACTION

LOW
01 02 03
04 05 06
07 08 09
10 11 12 HIGH

LUNCH TIME: _____

FOOD & DRINK

INTENSITY/REACTION

LOW
01 02 03
04 05 06
07 08 09
10 11 12 HIGH

DINNER TIME: _____

FOOD & DRINK

INTENSITY/REACTION

LOW
01 02 03
04 05 06
07 08 09
10 11 12 HIGH

SYMPTOMS -

PAIN MEASUREMENT SCALE

0 1 2 3 4 5 6 7 8 9 10

No Pain | Mild | Moderate | Severe | Very Severe | Worst Pain Possible

WATER TRACKER
1 2 3 4
5 6 7 8

STRESS LEVEL

BRISTOL STOOL CHART

TYPE 1 – HARD LUMPS ☐

TYPE 2 – LUMPY ☐

TYPE 3 – CRACKED ☐

TYPE 4 – SMOOTH ☐

TYPE 5 – SOFT BLOBS ☐

TYPE 6 – MUSHY EDGES ☐

TYPE 7 – JUST LIQUID ☐

NOTES

Daily IBS Diary

Date: ....

BREAKFAST TIME: _____

LUNCH TIME: _____

DINNER TIME: _____

FOOD & DRINK

INTENSITY/REACTION

LOW
- 01, 02, 03
- 04, 05, 06
- 07, 08, 09
- 10, 11, 12
HIGH

FOOD & DRINK

INTENSITY/REACTION

LOW
- 01, 02, 03
- 04, 05, 06
- 07, 08, 09
- 10, 11, 12
HIGH

FOOD & DRINK

INTENSITY/REACTION

LOW
- 01, 02, 03
- 04, 05, 06
- 07, 08, 09
- 10, 11, 12
HIGH

SYMPTOMS -

PAIN MEASUREMENT SCALE

0 1 2 3 4 5 6 7 8 9 10

| No Pain | Mild | Moderate | Severe | Very Severe | Worst Pain Possible |

WATER TRACKER
1 2 3 4
5 6 7 8

STRESS LEVEL

BRISTOL STOOL CHART

TYPE 1 – HARD LUMPS ☐

TYPE 2 – LUMPY ☐

TYPE 3 – CRACKED ☐

TYPE 4 – SMOOTH ☐

TYPE 5 – SOFT BLOBS ☐

TYPE 6 – MUSHY EDGES ☐

TYPE 7 – JUST LIQUID ☐

NOTES

Daily IBS Diary

Date: ....

BREAKFAST TIME: _____

FOOD & DRINK

INTENSITY/REACTION

LOW
01 02 03
04 05 06
07 08 09
10 11 12
HIGH

LUNCH TIME: _____

FOOD & DRINK

INTENSITY/REACTION

LOW
01 02 03
04 05 06
07 08 09
10 11 12
HIGH

DINNER TIME: _____

FOOD & DRINK

INTENSITY/REACTION

LOW
01 02 03
04 05 06
07 08 09
10 11 12
HIGH

SYMPTOMS -

PAIN MEASUREMENT SCALE

0 1 2 3 4 5 6 7 8 9 10

| No Pain | Mild | Moderate | Severe | Very Severe | Worst Pain Possible |

WATER TRACKER

1 2 3 4
5 6 7 8

STRESS LEVEL

BRISTOL STOOL CHART

TYPE 1 – HARD LUMPS ☐

TYPE 2 – LUMPY ☐

TYPE 3 – CRACKED ☐

TYPE 4 – SMOOTH ☐

TYPE 5 – SOFT BLOBS ☐

TYPE 6 – MUSHY EDGES ☐

TYPE 7 – JUST LIQUID ☐

NOTES

Daily IBS Diary

Date: ....

BREAKFAST TIME: _____   **LUNCH TIME:** _____   **DINNER TIME:** _____

FOOD & DRINK

INTENSITY/REACTION

LOW
- 01 02 03
- 04 05 06
- 07 08 09
- 10 11 12
HIGH

(repeated for Breakfast, Lunch, Dinner)

SYMPTOMS -

PAIN MEASUREMENT SCALE

0 1 2 3 4 5 6 7 8 9 10

- No Pain
- Mild
- Moderate
- Severe
- Very Severe
- Worst Pain Possible

WATER TRACKER
1 2 3 4
5 6 7 8

STRESS LEVEL

BRISTOL STOOL CHART

- TYPE 1 – HARD LUMPS ☐
- TYPE 2 – LUMPY ☐
- TYPE 3 – CRACKED ☐
- TYPE 4 – SMOOTH ☐
- TYPE 5 – SOFT BLOBS ☐
- TYPE 6 – MUSHY EDGES ☐
- TYPE 7 – JUST LIQUID ☐

NOTES

Daily IBS Diary

Date: ....

BREAKFAST TIME: _____

FOOD & DRINK

INTENSITY/REACTION

LOW
01 02 03
04 05 06
07 08 09
10 11 12 HIGH

LUNCH TIME: _____

FOOD & DRINK

INTENSITY/REACTION

LOW
01 02 03
04 05 06
07 08 09
10 11 12 HIGH

DINNER TIME: _____

FOOD & DRINK

INTENSITY/REACTION

LOW
01 02 03
04 05 06
07 08 09
10 11 12 HIGH

SYMPTOMS -

PAIN MEASUREMENT SCALE

0 1 2 3 4 5 6 7 8 9 10

No Pain | Mild | Moderate | Severe | Very Severe | Worst Pain Possible

WATER TRACKER

1 2 3 4
5 6 7 8

STRESS LEVEL

BRISTOL STOOL CHART

TYPE 1 – HARD LUMPS ☐
TYPE 2 – LUMPY ☐
TYPE 3 – CRACKED ☐
TYPE 4 – SMOOTH ☐
TYPE 5 – SOFT BLOBS ☐
TYPE 6 – MUSHY EDGES ☐
TYPE 7 – JUST LIQUID ☐

NOTES

Daily IBS Diary

Date: ....

BREAKFAST TIME: _____

FOOD & DRINK

INTENSITY/REACTION

LOW
01 02 03
04 05 06
07 08 09
10 11 12
HIGH

LUNCH TIME: _____

FOOD & DRINK

INTENSITY/REACTION

LOW
01 02 03
04 05 06
07 08 09
10 11 12
HIGH

DINNER TIME: _____

FOOD & DRINK

INTENSITY/REACTION

LOW
01 02 03
04 05 06
07 08 09
10 11 12
HIGH

SYMPTOMS -

PAIN MEASUREMENT SCALE

0 1 2 3 4 5 6 7 8 9 10

No Pain | Mild | Moderate | Severe | Very Severe | Worst Pain Possible

WATER TRACKER

1 2 3 4
5 6 7 8

STRESS LEVEL

BRISTOL STOOL CHART

TYPE 1 - HARD LUMPS ☐

TYPE 2 - LUMPY ☐

TYPE 3 - CRACKED ☐

TYPE 4 - SMOOTH ☐

TYPE 5 - SOFT BLOBS ☐

TYPE 6 - MUSHY EDGES ☐

TYPE 7 - JUST LIQUID ☐

NOTES

Daily IBS Diary

Date: ....

BREAKFAST TIME: _____

FOOD & DRINK

INTENSITY/REACTION

LOW 01 02 03
04 05 06
07 08 09
10 11 12 HIGH

LUNCH TIME: _____

FOOD & DRINK

INTENSITY/REACTION

LOW 01 02 03
04 05 06
07 08 09
10 11 12 HIGH

DINNER TIME: _____

FOOD & DRINK

INTENSITY/REACTION

LOW 01 02 03
04 05 06
07 08 09
10 11 12 HIGH

SYMPTOMS -

PAIN MEASUREMENT SCALE

0 1 2 3 4 5 6 7 8 9 10

No Pain | Mild | Moderate | Severe | Very Severe | Worst Pain Possible

WATER TRACKER

1 2 3 4
5 6 7 8

STRESS LEVEL

BRISTOL STOOL CHART

TYPE 1 – HARD LUMPS ☐

TYPE 2 – LUMPY ☐

TYPE 3 – CRACKED ☐

TYPE 4 – SMOOTH ☐

TYPE 5 – SOFT BLOBS ☐

TYPE 6 – MUSHY EDGES ☐

TYPE 7 – JUST LIQUID ☐

NOTES

Daily IBS Diary

Date: ....

BREAKFAST TIME: _____   LUNCH TIME: _____   DINNER TIME: _____

FOOD & DRINK

INTENSITY/REACTION

LOW 01 02 03
     04 05 06
     07 08 09
     10 11 12 HIGH

(Repeated for Breakfast, Lunch, and Dinner)

SYMPTOMS -

PAIN MEASUREMENT SCALE

0 1 2 3 4 5 6 7 8 9 10

No Pain — Mild — Moderate — Severe — Very Severe — Worst Pain Possible

WATER TRACKER
1 2 3 4
5 6 7 8

STRESS LEVEL

BRISTOL STOOL CHART

- TYPE 1 – HARD LUMPS ☐
- TYPE 2 – LUMPY ☐
- TYPE 3 – CRACKED ☐
- TYPE 4 – SMOOTH ☐
- TYPE 5 – SOFT BLOBS ☐
- TYPE 6 – MUSHY EDGES ☐
- TYPE 7 – JUST LIQUID ☐

NOTES

Daily IBS Diary

Date: ....

BREAKFAST TIME: _____

LUNCH TIME: _____

DINNER TIME: _____

FOOD & DRINK (Breakfast)

INTENSITY/REACTION
LOW 01 02 03 04 05 06 07 08 09 10 11 12 HIGH

FOOD & DRINK (Lunch)

INTENSITY/REACTION
LOW 01 02 03 04 05 06 07 08 09 10 11 12 HIGH

FOOD & DRINK (Dinner)

INTENSITY/REACTION
LOW 01 02 03 04 05 06 07 08 09 10 11 12 HIGH

SYMPTOMS -

PAIN MEASUREMENT SCALE
0 1 2 3 4 5 6 7 8 9 10

No Pain | Mild | Moderate | Severe | Very Severe | Worst Pain Possible

WATER TRACKER
1 2 3 4
5 6 7 8

STRESS LEVEL

BRISTOL STOOL CHART

- TYPE 1 – HARD LUMPS ☐
- TYPE 2 – LUMPY ☐
- TYPE 3 – CRACKED ☐
- TYPE 4 – SMOOTH ☐
- TYPE 5 – SOFT BLOBS ☐
- TYPE 6 – MUSHY EDGES ☐
- TYPE 7 – JUST LIQUID ☐

NOTES

Daily IBS Diary

Date: ....

BREAKFAST TIME: _____

FOOD & DRINK

INTENSITY/REACTION

LOW
01 02 03
04 05 06
07 08 09
10 11 12 HIGH

LUNCH TIME: _____

FOOD & DRINK

INTENSITY/REACTION

LOW
01 02 03
04 05 06
07 08 09
10 11 12 HIGH

DINNER TIME: _____

FOOD & DRINK

INTENSITY/REACTION

LOW
01 02 03
04 05 06
07 08 09
10 11 12 HIGH

SYMPTOMS -

PAIN MEASUREMENT SCALE

0 1 2 3 4 5 6 7 8 9 10

No Pain | Mild | Moderate | Severe | Very Severe | Worst Pain Possible

WATER TRACKER

1 2 3 4
5 6 7 8

STRESS LEVEL

BRISTOL STOOL CHART

TYPE 1 – HARD LUMPS ☐

TYPE 2 – LUMPY ☐

TYPE 3 – CRACKED ☐

TYPE 4 – SMOOTH ☐

TYPE 5 – SOFT BLOBS ☐

TYPE 6 – MUSHY EDGES ☐

TYPE 7 – JUST LIQUID ☐

NOTES

Daily IBS Diary

Date: ....

BREAKFAST TIME: _____

FOOD & DRINK

INTENSITY/REACTION

LOW
01 02 03
04 05 06
07 08 09
10 11 12   HIGH

LUNCH TIME: _____

FOOD & DRINK

INTENSITY/REACTION

LOW
01 02 03
04 05 06
07 08 09
10 11 12   HIGH

DINNER TIME: _____

FOOD & DRINK

INTENSITY/REACTION

LOW
01 02 03
04 05 06
07 08 09
10 11 12   HIGH

SYMPTOMS -

PAIN MEASUREMENT SCALE

0 1 2 3 4 5 6 7 8 9 10

No Pain | Mild | Moderate | Severe | Very Severe | Worst Pain Possible

WATER TRACKER

1 2 3 4
5 6 7 8

STRESS LEVEL

BRISTOL STOOL CHART

TYPE 1 – HARD LUMPS ☐

TYPE 2 – LUMPY ☐

TYPE 3 – CRACKED ☐

TYPE 4 – SMOOTH ☐

TYPE 5 – SOFT BLOBS ☐

TYPE 6 – MUSHY EDGES ☐

TYPE 7 – JUST LIQUID ☐

NOTES

Daily IBS Diary

Date: ....

BREAKFAST TIME: _____

FOOD & DRINK

INTENSITY/REACTION

LOW 01 02 03
     04 05 06
     07 08 09
     10 11 12 HIGH

LUNCH TIME: _____

FOOD & DRINK

INTENSITY/REACTION

LOW 01 02 03
     04 05 06
     07 08 09
     10 11 12 HIGH

DINNER TIME: _____

FOOD & DRINK

INTENSITY/REACTION

LOW 01 02 03
     04 05 06
     07 08 09
     10 11 12 HIGH

SYMPTOMS -

PAIN MEASUREMENT SCALE

0 1 2 3 4 5 6 7 8 9 10

No Pain | Mild | Moderate | Severe | Very Severe | Worst Pain Possible

WATER TRACKER

1 2 3 4
5 6 7 8

STRESS LEVEL

BRISTOL STOOL CHART

TYPE 1 – HARD LUMPS ☐
TYPE 2 – LUMPY ☐
TYPE 3 – CRACKED ☐
TYPE 4 – SMOOTH ☐
TYPE 5 – SOFT BLOBS ☐
TYPE 6 – MUSHY EDGES ☐
TYPE 7 – JUST LIQUID ☐

NOTES

Daily IBS Diary

Date: ....

BREAKFAST TIME: _____

FOOD & DRINK

INTENSITY/REACTION

LOW ‹01 ‹02 ‹03
‹04 ‹05 ‹06
‹07 ‹08 ‹09
‹10 ‹11 ‹12 HIGH

LUNCH TIME: _____

FOOD & DRINK

INTENSITY/REACTION

LOW ‹01 ‹02 ‹03
‹04 ‹05 ‹06
‹07 ‹08 ‹09
‹10 ‹11 ‹12 HIGH

DINNER TIME: _____

FOOD & DRINK

INTENSITY/REACTION

LOW ‹01 ‹02 ‹03
‹04 ‹05 ‹06
‹07 ‹08 ‹09
‹10 ‹11 ‹12 HIGH

SYMPTOMS -

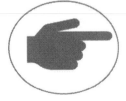

PAIN MEASUREMENT SCALE

0 1 2 3 4 5 6 7 8 9 10

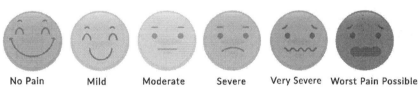

No Pain   Mild   Moderate   Severe   Very Severe   Worst Pain Possible

WATER TRACKER

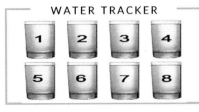

STRESS LEVEL

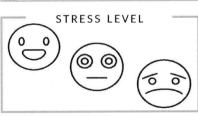

BRISTOL STOOL CHART

TYPE 1 – HARD LUMPS ☐

TYPE 2 – LUMPY ☐

TYPE 3 – CRACKED ☐

TYPE 4 – SMOOTH ☐

TYPE 5 – SOFT BLOBS ☐

TYPE 6 – MUSHY EDGES ☐

TYPE 7 – JUST LIQUID ☐

NOTES

Daily IBS Diary

Date: ....

BREAKFAST TIME: _____

LUNCH TIME: _____

DINNER TIME: _____

FOOD & DRINK

INTENSITY/REACTION

LOW
01 02 03
04 05 06
07 08 09
10 11 12 HIGH

FOOD & DRINK

INTENSITY/REACTION

LOW
01 02 03
04 05 06
07 08 09
10 11 12 HIGH

FOOD & DRINK

INTENSITY/REACTION

LOW
01 02 03
04 05 06
07 08 09
10 11 12 HIGH

SYMPTOMS -

PAIN MEASUREMENT SCALE

0 1 2 3 4 5 6 7 8 9 10

No Pain | Mild | Moderate | Severe | Very Severe | Worst Pain Possible

WATER TRACKER
1 2 3 4
5 6 7 8

STRESS LEVEL

BRISTOL STOOL CHART

TYPE 1 – HARD LUMPS ☐

TYPE 2 – LUMPY ☐

TYPE 3 – CRACKED ☐

TYPE 4 – SMOOTH ☐

TYPE 5 – SOFT BLOBS ☐

TYPE 6 – MUSHY EDGES ☐

TYPE 7 – JUST LIQUID ☐

NOTES

Daily IBS Diary

Date: ....

BREAKFAST TIME: _____

FOOD & DRINK

INTENSITY/REACTION

LOW — 01 02 03 04 05 06 07 08 09 10 11 12 HIGH

LUNCH TIME: _____

FOOD & DRINK

INTENSITY/REACTION

LOW — 01 02 03 04 05 06 07 08 09 10 11 12 HIGH

DINNER TIME: _____

FOOD & DRINK

INTENSITY/REACTION

LOW — 01 02 03 04 05 06 07 08 09 10 11 12 HIGH

SYMPTOMS -

PAIN MEASUREMENT SCALE

0 1 2 3 4 5 6 7 8 9 10

No Pain — Mild — Moderate — Severe — Very Severe — Worst Pain Possible

WATER TRACKER
1 2 3 4
5 6 7 8

STRESS LEVEL

BRISTOL STOOL CHART

TYPE 1 – HARD LUMPS ☐

TYPE 2 – LUMPY ☐

TYPE 3 – CRACKED ☐

TYPE 4 – SMOOTH ☐

TYPE 5 – SOFT BLOBS ☐

TYPE 6 – MUSHY EDGES ☐

TYPE 7 – JUST LIQUID ☐

NOTES

Daily IBS Diary

Date: ....

BREAKFAST TIME: _____

FOOD & DRINK

INTENSITY/REACTION

LOW 01 02 03
04 05 06
07 08 09
10 11 12 HIGH

LUNCH TIME: _____

FOOD & DRINK

INTENSITY/REACTION

LOW 01 02 03
04 05 06
07 08 09
10 11 12 HIGH

DINNER TIME: _____

FOOD & DRINK

INTENSITY/REACTION

LOW 01 02 03
04 05 06
07 08 09
10 11 12 HIGH

SYMPTOMS -

PAIN MEASUREMENT SCALE

0 1 2 3 4 5 6 7 8 9 10

No Pain — Mild — Moderate — Severe — Very Severe — Worst Pain Possible

WATER TRACKER
1 2 3 4
5 6 7 8

STRESS LEVEL

BRISTOL STOOL CHART

TYPE 1 – HARD LUMPS ☐
TYPE 2 – LUMPY ☐
TYPE 3 – CRACKED ☐
TYPE 4 – SMOOTH ☐
TYPE 5 – SOFT BLOBS ☐
TYPE 6 – MUSHY EDGES ☐
TYPE 7 – JUST LIQUID ☐

NOTES

Daily IBS Diary

Date: ....

BREAKFAST TIME: _____

FOOD & DRINK

INTENSITY/REACTION
LOW
01 02 03
04 05 06
07 08 09
10 11 12 HIGH

LUNCH TIME: _____

FOOD & DRINK

INTENSITY/REACTION
LOW
01 02 03
04 05 06
07 08 09
10 11 12 HIGH

DINNER TIME: _____

FOOD & DRINK

INTENSITY/REACTION
LOW
01 02 03
04 05 06
07 08 09
10 11 12 HIGH

SYMPTOMS -

PAIN MEASUREMENT SCALE

0 1 2 3 4 5 6 7 8 9 10

| No Pain | Mild | Moderate | Severe | Very Severe | Worst Pain Possible |

WATER TRACKER
1 2 3 4
5 6 7 8

STRESS LEVEL

BRISTOL STOOL CHART

TYPE 1 – HARD LUMPS ☐

TYPE 2 – LUMPY ☐

TYPE 3 – CRACKED ☐

TYPE 4 – SMOOTH ☐

TYPE 5 – SOFT BLOBS ☐

TYPE 6 – MUSHY EDGES ☐

TYPE 7 – JUST LIQUID ☐

NOTES

Daily IBS Diary

Date: ....

BREAKFAST TIME: _____

LUNCH TIME: _____

DINNER TIME: _____

FOOD & DRINK

INTENSITY/REACTION

LOW 01 02 03 04 05 06 07 08 09 10 11 12 HIGH

FOOD & DRINK

INTENSITY/REACTION

LOW 01 02 03 04 05 06 07 08 09 10 11 12 HIGH

FOOD & DRINK

INTENSITY/REACTION

LOW 01 02 03 04 05 06 07 08 09 10 11 12 HIGH

SYMPTOMS -

PAIN MEASUREMENT SCALE

0 1 2 3 4 5 6 7 8 9 10

No Pain — Mild — Moderate — Severe — Very Severe — Worst Pain Possible

WATER TRACKER

1 2 3 4
5 6 7 8

STRESS LEVEL

BRISTOL STOOL CHART

TYPE 1 – HARD LUMPS ☐

TYPE 2 – LUMPY ☐

TYPE 3 – CRACKED ☐

TYPE 4 – SMOOTH ☐

TYPE 5 – SOFT BLOBS ☐

TYPE 6 – MUSHY EDGES ☐

TYPE 7 – JUST LIQUID ☐

NOTES

Daily IBS Diary

Date: ....

BREAKFAST TIME: _____

FOOD & DRINK

INTENSITY/REACTION

LOW 01 02 03 04 05 06 07 08 09 10 11 12 HIGH

LUNCH TIME: _____

FOOD & DRINK

INTENSITY/REACTION

LOW 01 02 03 04 05 06 07 08 09 10 11 12 HIGH

DINNER TIME: _____

FOOD & DRINK

INTENSITY/REACTION

LOW 01 02 03 04 05 06 07 08 09 10 11 12 HIGH

SYMPTOMS -

PAIN MEASUREMENT SCALE

0 1 2 3 4 5 6 7 8 9 10

No Pain | Mild | Moderate | Severe | Very Severe | Worst Pain Possible

WATER TRACKER

1 2 3 4
5 6 7 8

STRESS LEVEL

BRISTOL STOOL CHART

TYPE 1 – HARD LUMPS ☐
TYPE 2 – LUMPY ☐
TYPE 3 – CRACKED ☐
TYPE 4 – SMOOTH ☐
TYPE 5 – SOFT BLOBS ☐
TYPE 6 – MUSHY EDGES ☐
TYPE 7 – JUST LIQUID ☐

NOTES

Daily IBS Diary

Date: ....

BREAKFAST TIME: _____

FOOD & DRINK

INTENSITY/REACTION

LOW
01 02 03
04 05 06
07 08 09
10 11 12
HIGH

LUNCH TIME: _____

FOOD & DRINK

INTENSITY/REACTION

LOW
01 02 03
04 05 06
07 08 09
10 11 12
HIGH

DINNER TIME: _____

FOOD & DRINK

INTENSITY/REACTION

LOW
01 02 03
04 05 06
07 08 09
10 11 12
HIGH

SYMPTOMS -

PAIN MEASUREMENT SCALE

0 1 2 3 4 5 6 7 8 9 10

No Pain | Mild | Moderate | Severe | Very Severe | Worst Pain Possible

WATER TRACKER
1 2 3 4
5 6 7 8

STRESS LEVEL

BRISTOL STOOL CHART

TYPE 1 - HARD LUMPS ☐

TYPE 2 - LUMPY ☐

TYPE 3 - CRACKED ☐

TYPE 4 - SMOOTH ☐

TYPE 5 - SOFT BLOBS ☐

TYPE 6 - MUSHY EDGES ☐

TYPE 7 - JUST LIQUID ☐

NOTES

Daily IBS Diary

Date: ....

BREAKFAST TIME: _____

FOOD & DRINK

INTENSITY/REACTION

LOW 01 02 03
04 05 06
07 08 09
10 11 12 HIGH

LUNCH TIME: _____

FOOD & DRINK

INTENSITY/REACTION

LOW 01 02 03
04 05 06
07 08 09
10 11 12 HIGH

DINNER TIME: _____

FOOD & DRINK

INTENSITY/REACTION

LOW 01 02 03
04 05 06
07 08 09
10 11 12 HIGH

SYMPTOMS -

PAIN MEASUREMENT SCALE

0 1 2 3 4 5 6 7 8 9 10

No Pain | Mild | Moderate | Severe | Very Severe | Worst Pain Possible

WATER TRACKER

1 2 3 4
5 6 7 8

STRESS LEVEL

BRISTOL STOOL CHART

TYPE 1 – HARD LUMPS
TYPE 2 – LUMPY
TYPE 3 – CRACKED
TYPE 4 – SMOOTH
TYPE 5 – SOFT BLOBS
TYPE 6 – MUSHY EDGES
TYPE 7 – JUST LIQUID

NOTES

Daily IBS Diary

Date: ....

BREAKFAST TIME: _____

FOOD & DRINK

INTENSITY/REACTION

LOW 01 02 03
04 05 06
07 08 09
10 11 12 HIGH

LUNCH TIME: _____

FOOD & DRINK

INTENSITY/REACTION

LOW 01 02 03
04 05 06
07 08 09
10 11 12 HIGH

DINNER TIME: _____

FOOD & DRINK

INTENSITY/REACTION

LOW 01 02 03
04 05 06
07 08 09
10 11 12 HIGH

SYMPTOMS -

PAIN MEASUREMENT SCALE

0 1 2 3 4 5 6 7 8 9 10

No Pain | Mild | Moderate | Severe | Very Severe | Worst Pain Possible

WATER TRACKER

1 2 3 4
5 6 7 8

STRESS LEVEL

BRISTOL STOOL CHART

TYPE 1 – HARD LUMPS ☐
TYPE 2 – LUMPY ☐
TYPE 3 – CRACKED ☐
TYPE 4 – SMOOTH ☐
TYPE 5 – SOFT BLOBS ☐
TYPE 6 – MUSHY EDGES ☐
TYPE 7 – JUST LIQUID ☐

NOTES

Daily IBS Diary

Date: ....

BREAKFAST TIME: _____

FOOD & DRINK

INTENSITY/REACTION

LOW
01 02 03
04 05 06
07 08 09
10 11 12 HIGH

LUNCH TIME: _____

FOOD & DRINK

INTENSITY/REACTION

LOW
01 02 03
04 05 06
07 08 09
10 11 12 HIGH

DINNER TIME: _____

FOOD & DRINK

INTENSITY/REACTION

LOW
01 02 03
04 05 06
07 08 09
10 11 12 HIGH

SYMPTOMS -

PAIN MEASUREMENT SCALE

0 1 2 3 4 5 6 7 8 9 10

No Pain | Mild | Moderate | Severe | Very Severe | Worst Pain Possible

WATER TRACKER
1 2 3 4
5 6 7 8

STRESS LEVEL

BRISTOL STOOL CHART

TYPE 1 – HARD LUMPS ☐

TYPE 2 – LUMPY ☐

TYPE 3 – CRACKED ☐

TYPE 4 – SMOOTH ☐

TYPE 5 – SOFT BLOBS ☐

TYPE 6 – MUSHY EDGES ☐

TYPE 7 – JUST LIQUID ☐

NOTES

Daily IBS Diary

Date: ....

BREAKFAST TIME: _____

FOOD & DRINK

INTENSITY/REACTION

LOW
- 01 02 03
- 04 05 06
- 07 08 09
- 10 11 12 HIGH

LUNCH TIME: _____

FOOD & DRINK

INTENSITY/REACTION

LOW
- 01 02 03
- 04 05 06
- 07 08 09
- 10 11 12 HIGH

DINNER TIME: _____

FOOD & DRINK

INTENSITY/REACTION

LOW
- 01 02 03
- 04 05 06
- 07 08 09
- 10 11 12 HIGH

SYMPTOMS -

PAIN MEASUREMENT SCALE

0 1 2 3 4 5 6 7 8 9 10

No Pain | Mild | Moderate | Severe | Very Severe | Worst Pain Possible

WATER TRACKER
1 2 3 4
5 6 7 8

STRESS LEVEL

BRISTOL STOOL CHART

- TYPE 1 – HARD LUMPS ☐
- TYPE 2 – LUMPY ☐
- TYPE 3 – CRACKED ☐
- TYPE 4 – SMOOTH ☐
- TYPE 5 – SOFT BLOBS ☐
- TYPE 6 – MUSHY EDGES ☐
- TYPE 7 – JUST LIQUID ☐

NOTES

Daily IBS Diary

Date: ....

BREAKFAST TIME: _____

FOOD & DRINK

INTENSITY/REACTION

LOW
01 02 03
04 05 06
07 08 09
10 11 12
HIGH

LUNCH TIME: _____

FOOD & DRINK

INTENSITY/REACTION

LOW
01 02 03
04 05 06
07 08 09
10 11 12
HIGH

DINNER TIME: _____

FOOD & DRINK

INTENSITY/REACTION

LOW
01 02 03
04 05 06
07 08 09
10 11 12
HIGH

SYMPTOMS -

PAIN MEASUREMENT SCALE

0 1 2 3 4 5 6 7 8 9 10

No Pain | Mild | Moderate | Severe | Very Severe | Worst Pain Possible

WATER TRACKER

1 2 3 4
5 6 7 8

STRESS LEVEL

BRISTOL STOOL CHART

TYPE 1 – HARD LUMPS ☐

TYPE 2 – LUMPY ☐

TYPE 3 – CRACKED ☐

TYPE 4 – SMOOTH ☐

TYPE 5 – SOFT BLOBS ☐

TYPE 6 – MUSHY EDGES ☐

TYPE 7 – JUST LIQUID ☐

NOTES

Daily IBS Diary

Date: ....

BREAKFAST TIME: _____

FOOD & DRINK

INTENSITY/REACTION

LOW 01 02 03
04 05 06
07 08 09
10 11 12 HIGH

LUNCH TIME: _____

FOOD & DRINK

INTENSITY/REACTION

LOW 01 02 03
04 05 06
07 08 09
10 11 12 HIGH

DINNER TIME: _____

FOOD & DRINK

INTENSITY/REACTION

LOW 01 02 03
04 05 06
07 08 09
10 11 12 HIGH

SYMPTOMS -

PAIN MEASUREMENT SCALE

0 1 2 3 4 5 6 7 8 9 10

No Pain | Mild | Moderate | Severe | Very Severe | Worst Pain Possible

WATER TRACKER

1 2 3 4
5 6 7 8

STRESS LEVEL

BRISTOL STOOL CHART

TYPE 1 – HARD LUMPS ☐

TYPE 2 – LUMPY ☐

TYPE 3 – CRACKED ☐

TYPE 4 – SMOOTH ☐

TYPE 5 – SOFT BLOBS ☐

TYPE 6 – MUSHY EDGES ☐

TYPE 7 – JUST LIQUID ☐

NOTES

Daily IBS Diary

Date: ....

BREAKFAST TIME: _____

FOOD & DRINK

INTENSITY/REACTION

LOW
01 02 03
04 05 06
07 08 09
10 11 12
HIGH

LUNCH TIME: _____

FOOD & DRINK

INTENSITY/REACTION

LOW
01 02 03
04 05 06
07 08 09
10 11 12
HIGH

DINNER TIME: _____

FOOD & DRINK

INTENSITY/REACTION

LOW
01 02 03
04 05 06
07 08 09
10 11 12
HIGH

SYMPTOMS -

PAIN MEASUREMENT SCALE

0 1 2 3 4 5 6 7 8 9 10

No Pain | Mild | Moderate | Severe | Very Severe | Worst Pain Possible

WATER TRACKER

1 2 3 4
5 6 7 8

STRESS LEVEL

BRISTOL STOOL CHART

TYPE 1 – HARD LUMPS ☐

TYPE 2 – LUMPY ☐

TYPE 3 – CRACKED ☐

TYPE 4 – SMOOTH ☐

TYPE 5 – SOFT BLOBS ☐

TYPE 6 – MUSHY EDGES ☐

TYPE 7 – JUST LIQUID ☐

NOTES

Daily IBS Diary

Date: ....

BREAKFAST TIME: ....

LUNCH TIME: ....

DINNER TIME: ....

FOOD & DRINK

INTENSITY/REACTION

LOW 01 02 03 04 05 06 07 08 09 10 11 12 HIGH

FOOD & DRINK

INTENSITY/REACTION

LOW 01 02 03 04 05 06 07 08 09 10 11 12 HIGH

FOOD & DRINK

INTENSITY/REACTION

LOW 01 02 03 04 05 06 07 08 09 10 11 12 HIGH

SYMPTOMS -

PAIN MEASUREMENT SCALE

0 1 2 3 4 5 6 7 8 9 10

No Pain | Mild | Moderate | Severe | Very Severe | Worst Pain Possible

WATER TRACKER
1 2 3 4 5 6 7 8

STRESS LEVEL

BRISTOL STOOL CHART

TYPE 1 – HARD LUMPS ☐

TYPE 2 – LUMPY ☐

TYPE 3 – CRACKED ☐

TYPE 4 – SMOOTH ☐

TYPE 5 – SOFT BLOBS ☐

TYPE 6 – MUSHY EDGES ☐

TYPE 7 – JUST LIQUID ☐

NOTES

Daily IBS Diary

Date: ....

BREAKFAST TIME: _____

FOOD & DRINK

INTENSITY/REACTION

LOW
01 02 03
04 05 06
07 08 09
10 11 12 HIGH

LUNCH TIME: _____

FOOD & DRINK

INTENSITY/REACTION

LOW
01 02 03
04 05 06
07 08 09
10 11 12 HIGH

DINNER TIME: _____

FOOD & DRINK

INTENSITY/REACTION

LOW
01 02 03
04 05 06
07 08 09
10 11 12 HIGH

SYMPTOMS -

PAIN MEASUREMENT SCALE

0 1 2 3 4 5 6 7 8 9 10

No Pain | Mild | Moderate | Severe | Very Severe | Worst Pain Possible

WATER TRACKER

1 2 3 4
5 6 7 8

STRESS LEVEL

BRISTOL STOOL CHART

TYPE 1 – HARD LUMPS ☐

TYPE 2 – LUMPY ☐

TYPE 3 – CRACKED ☐

TYPE 4 – SMOOTH ☐

TYPE 5 – SOFT BLOBS ☐

TYPE 6 – MUSHY EDGES ☐

TYPE 7 – JUST LIQUID ☐

NOTES

Daily IBS Diary

Date: ....

BREAKFAST TIME: _____

LUNCH TIME: _____

DINNER TIME: _____

FOOD & DRINK

INTENSITY/REACTION

LOW
01 02 03
04 05 06
07 08 09
10 11 12
HIGH

FOOD & DRINK

INTENSITY/REACTION

LOW
01 02 03
04 05 06
07 08 09
10 11 12
HIGH

FOOD & DRINK

INTENSITY/REACTION

LOW
01 02 03
04 05 06
07 08 09
10 11 12
HIGH

SYMPTOMS -

PAIN MEASUREMENT SCALE

0 1 2 3 4 5 6 7 8 9 10

No Pain | Mild | Moderate | Severe | Very Severe | Worst Pain Possible

WATER TRACKER

1 2 3 4
5 6 7 8

STRESS LEVEL

BRISTOL STOOL CHART

TYPE 1 – HARD LUMPS ☐

TYPE 2 – LUMPY ☐

TYPE 3 – CRACKED ☐

TYPE 4 – SMOOTH ☐

TYPE 5 – SOFT BLOBS ☐

TYPE 6 – MUSHY EDGES ☐

TYPE 7 – JUST LIQUID ☐

NOTES

Daily IBS Diary

Date: ....

BREAKFAST TIME: _____

FOOD & DRINK

INTENSITY/REACTION

LOW
- 01
- 02
- 03
- 04
- 05
- 06
- 07
- 08
- 09
- 10
- 11
- 12

HIGH

LUNCH TIME: _____

FOOD & DRINK

INTENSITY/REACTION

LOW
- 01
- 02
- 03
- 04
- 05
- 06
- 07
- 08
- 09
- 10
- 11
- 12

HIGH

DINNER TIME: _____

FOOD & DRINK

INTENSITY/REACTION

LOW
- 01
- 02
- 03
- 04
- 05
- 06
- 07
- 08
- 09
- 10
- 11
- 12

HIGH

SYMPTOMS -

PAIN MEASUREMENT SCALE

0 1 2 3 4 5 6 7 8 9 10

| No Pain | Mild | Moderate | Severe | Very Severe | Worst Pain Possible |

WATER TRACKER

1 2 3 4
5 6 7 8

STRESS LEVEL

BRISTOL STOOL CHART

- TYPE 1 – HARD LUMPS ☐
- TYPE 2 – LUMPY ☐
- TYPE 3 – CRACKED ☐
- TYPE 4 – SMOOTH ☐
- TYPE 5 – SOFT BLOBS ☐
- TYPE 6 – MUSHY EDGES ☐
- TYPE 7 – JUST LIQUID ☐

NOTES

Daily IBS Diary

Date: ....

BREAKFAST TIME: _____

FOOD & DRINK

INTENSITY/REACTION

LOW
01 02 03
04 05 06
07 08 09
10 11 12
HIGH

LUNCH TIME: _____

FOOD & DRINK

INTENSITY/REACTION

LOW
01 02 03
04 05 06
07 08 09
10 11 12
HIGH

DINNER TIME: _____

FOOD & DRINK

INTENSITY/REACTION

LOW
01 02 03
04 05 06
07 08 09
10 11 12
HIGH

SYMPTOMS -

PAIN MEASUREMENT SCALE

0 1 2 3 4 5 6 7 8 9 10

No Pain | Mild | Moderate | Severe | Very Severe | Worst Pain Possible

WATER TRACKER
1 2 3 4
5 6 7 8

STRESS LEVEL

BRISTOL STOOL CHART

TYPE 1 – HARD LUMPS ☐

TYPE 2 – LUMPY ☐

TYPE 3 – CRACKED ☐

TYPE 4 – SMOOTH ☐

TYPE 5 – SOFT BLOBS ☐

TYPE 6 – MUSHY EDGES ☐

TYPE 7 – JUST LIQUID ☐

NOTES

Daily IBS Diary

Date: ....

BREAKFAST TIME: _____ LUNCH TIME: _____ DINNER TIME: _____

FOOD & DRINK

INTENSITY/REACTION

Breakfast:
LOW 01 02 03 04 05 06 07 08 09 10 11 12 HIGH

Lunch:
LOW 01 02 03 04 05 06 07 08 09 10 11 12 HIGH

Dinner:
LOW 01 02 03 04 05 06 07 08 09 10 11 12 HIGH

SYMPTOMS -

PAIN MEASUREMENT SCALE

0 1 2 3 4 5 6 7 8 9 10

No Pain | Mild | Moderate | Severe | Very Severe | Worst Pain Possible

WATER TRACKER

1 2 3 4
5 6 7 8

STRESS LEVEL

BRISTOL STOOL CHART

TYPE 1 – HARD LUMPS ☐

TYPE 2 – LUMPY ☐

TYPE 3 – CRACKED ☐

TYPE 4 – SMOOTH ☐

TYPE 5 – SOFT BLOBS ☐

TYPE 6 – MUSHY EDGES ☐

TYPE 7 – JUST LIQUID ☐

NOTES

Daily IBS Diary

Date: ....

BREAKFAST TIME: _____

FOOD & DRINK

INTENSITY/REACTION

LOW
01 02 03
04 05 06
07 08 09
10 11 12   HIGH

LUNCH TIME: _____

FOOD & DRINK

INTENSITY/REACTION

LOW
01 02 03
04 05 06
07 08 09
10 11 12   HIGH

DINNER TIME: _____

FOOD & DRINK

INTENSITY/REACTION

LOW
01 02 03
04 05 06
07 08 09
10 11 12   HIGH

SYMPTOMS -

PAIN MEASUREMENT SCALE

0 1 2 3 4 5 6 7 8 9 10

No Pain | Mild | Moderate | Severe | Very Severe | Worst Pain Possible

WATER TRACKER

1 2 3 4
5 6 7 8

STRESS LEVEL

BRISTOL STOOL CHART

TYPE 1 – HARD LUMPS ☐

TYPE 2 – LUMPY ☐

TYPE 3 – CRACKED ☐

TYPE 4 – SMOOTH ☐

TYPE 5 – SOFT BLOBS ☐

TYPE 6 – MUSHY EDGES ☐

TYPE 7 – JUST LIQUID ☐

NOTES

Daily IBS Diary

Date: ....

BREAKFAST TIME: _____

FOOD & DRINK

INTENSITY/REACTION
LOW 01 02 03 04 05 06 07 08 09 10 11 12 HIGH

LUNCH TIME: _____

FOOD & DRINK

INTENSITY/REACTION
LOW 01 02 03 04 05 06 07 08 09 10 11 12 HIGH

DINNER TIME: _____

FOOD & DRINK

INTENSITY/REACTION
LOW 01 02 03 04 05 06 07 08 09 10 11 12 HIGH

SYMPTOMS -

PAIN MEASUREMENT SCALE
0 1 2 3 4 5 6 7 8 9 10

No Pain | Mild | Moderate | Severe | Very Severe | Worst Pain Possible

WATER TRACKER
1 2 3 4 5 6 7 8

STRESS LEVEL

BRISTOL STOOL CHART
TYPE 1 – HARD LUMPS ☐
TYPE 2 – LUMPY ☐
TYPE 3 – CRACKED ☐
TYPE 4 – SMOOTH ☐
TYPE 5 – SOFT BLOBS ☐
TYPE 6 – MUSHY EDGES ☐
TYPE 7 – JUST LIQUID ☐

NOTES

Daily IBS Diary

Date: ....

BREAKFAST TIME: _____

FOOD & DRINK

INTENSITY/REACTION

LOW
01 02 03
04 05 06
07 08 09
10 11 12 HIGH

LUNCH TIME: _____

FOOD & DRINK

INTENSITY/REACTION

LOW
01 02 03
04 05 06
07 08 09
10 11 12 HIGH

DINNER TIME: _____

FOOD & DRINK

INTENSITY/REACTION

LOW
01 02 03
04 05 06
07 08 09
10 11 12 HIGH

SYMPTOMS -

PAIN MEASUREMENT SCALE

0 1 2 3 4 5 6 7 8 9 10

No Pain | Mild | Moderate | Severe | Very Severe | Worst Pain Possible

WATER TRACKER

1 2 3 4
5 6 7 8

STRESS LEVEL

BRISTOL STOOL CHART

TYPE 1 – HARD LUMPS ☐

TYPE 2 – LUMPY ☐

TYPE 3 – CRACKED ☐

TYPE 4 – SMOOTH ☐

TYPE 5 – SOFT BLOBS ☐

TYPE 6 – MUSHY EDGES ☐

TYPE 7 – JUST LIQUID ☐

NOTES

Daily IBS Diary

Date: ....

BREAKFAST TIME: _____

FOOD & DRINK

INTENSITY/REACTION
LOW 01 02 03
04 05 06
07 08 09
10 11 12 HIGH

LUNCH TIME: _____

FOOD & DRINK

INTENSITY/REACTION
LOW 01 02 03
04 05 06
07 08 09
10 11 12 HIGH

DINNER TIME: _____

FOOD & DRINK

INTENSITY/REACTION
LOW 01 02 03
04 05 06
07 08 09
10 11 12 HIGH

SYMPTOMS -

PAIN MEASUREMENT SCALE
0 1 2 3 4 5 6 7 8 9 10

No Pain | Mild | Moderate | Severe | Very Severe | Worst Pain Possible

WATER TRACKER
1 2 3 4
5 6 7 8

STRESS LEVEL

BRISTOL STOOL CHART

TYPE 1 – HARD LUMPS ☐
TYPE 2 – LUMPY ☐
TYPE 3 – CRACKED ☐
TYPE 4 – SMOOTH ☐
TYPE 5 – SOFT BLOBS ☐
TYPE 6 – MUSHY EDGES ☐
TYPE 7 – JUST LIQUID ☐

NOTES

Daily IBS Diary

Date: ....

BREAKFAST TIME: _____

FOOD & DRINK

INTENSITY/REACTION

LOW 01 02 03
04 05 06
07 08 09
10 11 12 HIGH

LUNCH TIME: _____

FOOD & DRINK

INTENSITY/REACTION

LOW 01 02 03
04 05 06
07 08 09
10 11 12 HIGH

DINNER TIME: _____

FOOD & DRINK

INTENSITY/REACTION

LOW 01 02 03
04 05 06
07 08 09
10 11 12 HIGH

SYMPTOMS -

PAIN MEASUREMENT SCALE

0 1 2 3 4 5 6 7 8 9 10

No Pain | Mild | Moderate | Severe | Very Severe | Worst Pain Possible

WATER TRACKER

1 2 3 4
5 6 7 8

STRESS LEVEL

BRISTOL STOOL CHART

TYPE 1 – HARD LUMPS ☐
TYPE 2 – LUMPY ☐
TYPE 3 – CRACKED ☐
TYPE 4 – SMOOTH ☐
TYPE 5 – SOFT BLOBS ☐
TYPE 6 – MUSHY EDGES ☐
TYPE 7 – JUST LIQUID ☐

NOTES

Daily IBS Diary

Date: ....

BREAKFAST TIME: _____

FOOD & DRINK

INTENSITY/REACTION

LOW 01 02 03
04 05 06
07 08 09
10 11 12 HIGH

LUNCH TIME: _____

FOOD & DRINK

INTENSITY/REACTION

LOW 01 02 03
04 05 06
07 08 09
10 11 12 HIGH

DINNER TIME: _____

FOOD & DRINK

INTENSITY/REACTION

LOW 01 02 03
04 05 06
07 08 09
10 11 12 HIGH

SYMPTOMS -

PAIN MEASUREMENT SCALE

0 1 2 3 4 5 6 7 8 9 10

No Pain | Mild | Moderate | Severe | Very Severe | Worst Pain Possible

WATER TRACKER

1 2 3 4
5 6 7 8

STRESS LEVEL

BRISTOL STOOL CHART

TYPE 1 – HARD LUMPS ☐
TYPE 2 – LUMPY ☐
TYPE 3 – CRACKED ☐
TYPE 4 – SMOOTH ☐
TYPE 5 – SOFT BLOBS ☐
TYPE 6 – MUSHY EDGES ☐
TYPE 7 – JUST LIQUID ☐

NOTES

Daily IBS Diary

Date: ....

BREAKFAST TIME: _____

FOOD & DRINK

INTENSITY/REACTION

LOW
01 02 03
04 05 06
07 08 09
10 11 12
HIGH

LUNCH TIME: _____

FOOD & DRINK

INTENSITY/REACTION

LOW
01 02 03
04 05 06
07 08 09
10 11 12
HIGH

DINNER TIME: _____

FOOD & DRINK

INTENSITY/REACTION

LOW
01 02 03
04 05 06
07 08 09
10 11 12
HIGH

SYMPTOMS -

PAIN MEASUREMENT SCALE

0 1 2 3 4 5 6 7 8 9 10

No Pain | Mild | Moderate | Severe | Very Severe | Worst Pain Possible

WATER TRACKER

1 2 3 4
5 6 7 8

STRESS LEVEL

BRISTOL STOOL CHART

TYPE 1 - HARD LUMPS ☐
TYPE 2 - LUMPY ☐
TYPE 3 - CRACKED ☐
TYPE 4 - SMOOTH ☐
TYPE 5 - SOFT BLOBS ☐
TYPE 6 - MUSHY EDGES ☐
TYPE 7 - JUST LIQUID ☐

NOTES

Daily IBS Diary

Date: ....

BREAKFAST TIME: _____

FOOD & DRINK

INTENSITY/REACTION

LOW 01 02 03
     04 05 06
     07 08 09
     10 11 12 HIGH

LUNCH TIME: _____

FOOD & DRINK

INTENSITY/REACTION

LOW 01 02 03
     04 05 06
     07 08 09
     10 11 12 HIGH

DINNER TIME: _____

FOOD & DRINK

INTENSITY/REACTION

LOW 01 02 03
     04 05 06
     07 08 09
     10 11 12 HIGH

SYMPTOMS -

PAIN MEASUREMENT SCALE

0 1 2 3 4 5 6 7 8 9 10

No Pain | Mild | Moderate | Severe | Very Severe | Worst Pain Possible

WATER TRACKER

1 2 3 4
5 6 7 8

STRESS LEVEL

BRISTOL STOOL CHART

TYPE 1 – HARD LUMPS ☐
TYPE 2 – LUMPY ☐
TYPE 3 – CRACKED ☐
TYPE 4 – SMOOTH ☐
TYPE 5 – SOFT BLOBS ☐
TYPE 6 – MUSHY EDGES ☐
TYPE 7 – JUST LIQUID ☐

NOTES

Daily IBS Diary

Date: ....

BREAKFAST TIME: _____

FOOD & DRINK

INTENSITY/REACTION

LOW 01 02 03 04 05 06 07 08 09 10 11 12 HIGH

LUNCH TIME: _____

FOOD & DRINK

INTENSITY/REACTION

LOW 01 02 03 04 05 06 07 08 09 10 11 12 HIGH

DINNER TIME: _____

FOOD & DRINK

INTENSITY/REACTION

LOW 01 02 03 04 05 06 07 08 09 10 11 12 HIGH

SYMPTOMS -

PAIN MEASUREMENT SCALE

0 1 2 3 4 5 6 7 8 9 10

No Pain | Mild | Moderate | Severe | Very Severe | Worst Pain Possible

WATER TRACKER
1 2 3 4
5 6 7 8

STRESS LEVEL

BRISTOL STOOL CHART

TYPE 1 – HARD LUMPS ☐

TYPE 2 – LUMPY ☐

TYPE 3 – CRACKED ☐

TYPE 4 – SMOOTH ☐

TYPE 5 – SOFT BLOBS ☐

TYPE 6 – MUSHY EDGES ☐

TYPE 7 – JUST LIQUID ☐

NOTES

Daily IBS Diary

Date: ....

BREAKFAST TIME: _____

FOOD & DRINK

INTENSITY/REACTION
LOW — 01, 02, 03, 04, 05, 06, 07, 08, 09, 10, 11, 12 — HIGH

LUNCH TIME: _____

FOOD & DRINK

INTENSITY/REACTION
LOW — 01, 02, 03, 04, 05, 06, 07, 08, 09, 10, 11, 12 — HIGH

DINNER TIME: _____

FOOD & DRINK

INTENSITY/REACTION
LOW — 01, 02, 03, 04, 05, 06, 07, 08, 09, 10, 11, 12 — HIGH

SYMPTOMS -

PAIN MEASUREMENT SCALE
0 1 2 3 4 5 6 7 8 9 10

No Pain | Mild | Moderate | Severe | Very Severe | Worst Pain Possible

WATER TRACKER
1 2 3 4
5 6 7 8

STRESS LEVEL

BRISTOL STOOL CHART

TYPE 1 – HARD LUMPS ☐
TYPE 2 – LUMPY ☐
TYPE 3 – CRACKED ☐
TYPE 4 – SMOOTH ☐
TYPE 5 – SOFT BLOBS ☐
TYPE 6 – MUSHY EDGES ☐
TYPE 7 – JUST LIQUID ☐

NOTES

Daily IBS Diary

Date: ....

BREAKFAST TIME: _____   **LUNCH TIME:** _____   **DINNER TIME:** _____

FOOD & DRINK

INTENSITY/REACTION

LOW
- 01 02 03
- 04 05 06
- 07 08 09
- 10 11 12
HIGH

FOOD & DRINK

INTENSITY/REACTION

LOW
- 01 02 03
- 04 05 06
- 07 08 09
- 10 11 12
HIGH

FOOD & DRINK

INTENSITY/REACTION

LOW
- 01 02 03
- 04 05 06
- 07 08 09
- 10 11 12
HIGH

SYMPTOMS -

PAIN MEASUREMENT SCALE

0 1 2 3 4 5 6 7 8 9 10

No Pain | Mild | Moderate | Severe | Very Severe | Worst Pain Possible

WATER TRACKER
1 2 3 4
5 6 7 8

STRESS LEVEL

BRISTOL STOOL CHART

TYPE 1 – HARD LUMPS ☐

TYPE 2 – LUMPY ☐

TYPE 3 – CRACKED ☐

TYPE 4 – SMOOTH ☐

TYPE 5 – SOFT BLOBS ☐

TYPE 6 – MUSHY EDGES ☐

TYPE 7 – JUST LIQUID ☐

NOTES

Daily IBS Diary

Date: ....

BREAKFAST TIME: _____

FOOD & DRINK

INTENSITY/REACTION

LOW 01 02 03
04 05 06
07 08 09
10 11 12 HIGH

LUNCH TIME: _____

FOOD & DRINK

INTENSITY/REACTION

LOW 01 02 03
04 05 06
07 08 09
10 11 12 HIGH

DINNER TIME: _____

FOOD & DRINK

INTENSITY/REACTION

LOW 01 02 03
04 05 06
07 08 09
10 11 12 HIGH

SYMPTOMS -

PAIN MEASUREMENT SCALE

0 1 2 3 4 5 6 7 8 9 10

No Pain | Mild | Moderate | Severe | Very Severe | Worst Pain Possible

WATER TRACKER

1 2 3 4
5 6 7 8

STRESS LEVEL

BRISTOL STOOL CHART

TYPE 1 – HARD LUMPS ☐
TYPE 2 – LUMPY ☐
TYPE 3 – CRACKED ☐
TYPE 4 – SMOOTH ☐
TYPE 5 – SOFT BLOBS ☐
TYPE 6 – MUSHY EDGES ☐
TYPE 7 – JUST LIQUID ☐

NOTES

Daily IBS Diary

Date: ....

BREAKFAST TIME: _____

FOOD & DRINK

INTENSITY/REACTION

LOW 01 02 03 04 05 06 07 08 09 10 11 12 HIGH

LUNCH TIME: _____

FOOD & DRINK

INTENSITY/REACTION

LOW 01 02 03 04 05 06 07 08 09 10 11 12 HIGH

DINNER TIME: _____

FOOD & DRINK

INTENSITY/REACTION

LOW 01 02 03 04 05 06 07 08 09 10 11 12 HIGH

SYMPTOMS -

PAIN MEASUREMENT SCALE

0 1 2 3 4 5 6 7 8 9 10

No Pain — Mild — Moderate — Severe — Very Severe — Worst Pain Possible

WATER TRACKER
1 2 3 4
5 6 7 8

STRESS LEVEL

BRISTOL STOOL CHART

TYPE 1 – HARD LUMPS ☐

TYPE 2 – LUMPY ☐

TYPE 3 – CRACKED ☐

TYPE 4 – SMOOTH ☐

TYPE 5 – SOFT BLOBS ☐

TYPE 6 – MUSHY EDGES ☐

TYPE 7 – JUST LIQUID ☐

NOTES

Daily IBS Diary

Date: ....

BREAKFAST TIME: ....

FOOD & DRINK

INTENSITY/REACTION

LOW
01 02 03
04 05 06
07 08 09
10 11 12
HIGH

LUNCH TIME: ....

FOOD & DRINK

INTENSITY/REACTION

LOW
01 02 03
04 05 06
07 08 09
10 11 12
HIGH

DINNER TIME: ....

FOOD & DRINK

INTENSITY/REACTION

LOW
01 02 03
04 05 06
07 08 09
10 11 12
HIGH

SYMPTOMS -

PAIN MEASUREMENT SCALE

0 1 2 3 4 5 6 7 8 9 10

No Pain | Mild | Moderate | Severe | Very Severe | Worst Pain Possible

WATER TRACKER

1 2 3 4
5 6 7 8

STRESS LEVEL

BRISTOL STOOL CHART

TYPE 1 – HARD LUMPS ☐
TYPE 2 – LUMPY ☐
TYPE 3 – CRACKED ☐
TYPE 4 – SMOOTH ☐
TYPE 5 – SOFT BLOBS ☐
TYPE 6 – MUSHY EDGES ☐
TYPE 7 – JUST LIQUID ☐

NOTES

Daily IBS Diary

Date: ....

BREAKFAST TIME: _____

LUNCH TIME: _____

DINNER TIME: _____

FOOD & DRINK

INTENSITY/REACTION

LOW
- 01 02 03
- 04 05 06
- 07 08 09
- 10 11 12
HIGH

FOOD & DRINK

INTENSITY/REACTION

LOW
- 01 02 03
- 04 05 06
- 07 08 09
- 10 11 12
HIGH

FOOD & DRINK

INTENSITY/REACTION

LOW
- 01 02 03
- 04 05 06
- 07 08 09
- 10 11 12
HIGH

SYMPTOMS -

PAIN MEASUREMENT SCALE

0 1 2 3 4 5 6 7 8 9 10

No Pain | Mild | Moderate | Severe | Very Severe | Worst Pain Possible

BRISTOL STOOL CHART

TYPE 1 – HARD LUMPS ☐

TYPE 2 – LUMPY ☐

TYPE 3 – CRACKED ☐

TYPE 4 – SMOOTH ☐

TYPE 5 – SOFT BLOBS ☐

TYPE 6 – MUSHY EDGES ☐

TYPE 7 – JUST LIQUID ☐

WATER TRACKER

1 2 3 4
5 6 7 8

STRESS LEVEL

NOTES

Daily IBS Diary

Date: ....

BREAKFAST TIME: _____

FOOD & DRINK

INTENSITY/REACTION
LOW
01 02 03
04 05 06
07 08 09
10 11 12 HIGH

LUNCH TIME: _____

FOOD & DRINK

INTENSITY/REACTION
LOW
01 02 03
04 05 06
07 08 09
10 11 12 HIGH

DINNER TIME: _____

FOOD & DRINK

INTENSITY/REACTION
LOW
01 02 03
04 05 06
07 08 09
10 11 12 HIGH

SYMPTOMS -

PAIN MEASUREMENT SCALE

0 1 2 3 4 5 6 7 8 9 10

No Pain | Mild | Moderate | Severe | Very Severe | Worst Pain Possible

WATER TRACKER
1 2 3 4
5 6 7 8

STRESS LEVEL

BRISTOL STOOL CHART

TYPE 1 – HARD LUMPS ☐
TYPE 2 – LUMPY ☐
TYPE 3 – CRACKED ☐
TYPE 4 – SMOOTH ☐
TYPE 5 – SOFT BLOBS ☐
TYPE 6 – MUSHY EDGES ☐
TYPE 7 – JUST LIQUID ☐

NOTES

Daily IBS Diary

Date: ....

BREAKFAST TIME: _____

FOOD & DRINK

INTENSITY/REACTION

LOW 01 02 03
04 05 06
07 08 09
10 11 12 HIGH

LUNCH TIME: _____

FOOD & DRINK

INTENSITY/REACTION

LOW 01 02 03
04 05 06
07 08 09
10 11 12 HIGH

DINNER TIME: _____

FOOD & DRINK

INTENSITY/REACTION

LOW 01 02 03
04 05 06
07 08 09
10 11 12 HIGH

SYMPTOMS -

PAIN MEASUREMENT SCALE

0 1 2 3 4 5 6 7 8 9 10

No Pain | Mild | Moderate | Severe | Very Severe | Worst Pain Possible

WATER TRACKER

1 2 3 4
5 6 7 8

STRESS LEVEL

BRISTOL STOOL CHART

TYPE 1 – HARD LUMPS ☐

TYPE 2 – LUMPY ☐

TYPE 3 – CRACKED ☐

TYPE 4 – SMOOTH ☐

TYPE 5 – SOFT BLOBS ☐

TYPE 6 – MUSHY EDGES ☐

TYPE 7 – JUST LIQUID ☐

NOTES

Daily IBS Diary

Date: ....

BREAKFAST TIME: _____

FOOD & DRINK

INTENSITY/REACTION

LOW 01 02 03 04 05 06 07 08 09 10 11 12 HIGH

LUNCH TIME: _____

FOOD & DRINK

INTENSITY/REACTION

LOW 01 02 03 04 05 06 07 08 09 10 11 12 HIGH

DINNER TIME: _____

FOOD & DRINK

INTENSITY/REACTION

LOW 01 02 03 04 05 06 07 08 09 10 11 12 HIGH

SYMPTOMS -

PAIN MEASUREMENT SCALE

0 1 2 3 4 5 6 7 8 9 10

No Pain | Mild | Moderate | Severe | Very Severe | Worst Pain Possible

WATER TRACKER
1 2 3 4
5 6 7 8

STRESS LEVEL

BRISTOL STOOL CHART

TYPE 1 - HARD LUMPS ☐

TYPE 2 - LUMPY ☐

TYPE 3 - CRACKED ☐

TYPE 4 - SMOOTH ☐

TYPE 5 - SOFT BLOBS ☐

TYPE 6 - MUSHY EDGES ☐

TYPE 7 - JUST LIQUID ☐

NOTES

Daily IBS Diary

Date: ....

BREAKFAST TIME: .... LUNCH TIME: .... DINNER TIME: ....

FOOD & DRINK

FOOD & DRINK

FOOD & DRINK

INTENSITY/REACTION

LOW 01 02 03
04 05 06
07 08 09
10 11 12 HIGH

INTENSITY/REACTION

LOW 01 02 03
04 05 06
07 08 09
10 11 12 HIGH

INTENSITY/REACTION

LOW 01 02 03
04 05 06
07 08 09
10 11 12 HIGH

SYMPTOMS -

PAIN MEASUREMENT SCALE

0 1 2 3 4 5 6 7 8 9 10

No Pain | Mild | Moderate | Severe | Very Severe | Worst Pain Possible

WATER TRACKER

1 2 3 4
5 6 7 8

STRESS LEVEL

BRISTOL STOOL CHART

TYPE 1 – HARD LUMPS ☐

TYPE 2 – LUMPY ☐

TYPE 3 – CRACKED ☐

TYPE 4 – SMOOTH ☐

TYPE 5 – SOFT BLOBS ☐

TYPE 6 – MUSHY EDGES ☐

TYPE 7 – JUST LIQUID ☐

NOTES

Daily IBS Diary

Date: ....

BREAKFAST TIME: _____

FOOD & DRINK

INTENSITY/REACTION

LOW
01 02 03
04 05 06
07 08 09
10 11 12
HIGH

LUNCH TIME: _____

FOOD & DRINK

INTENSITY/REACTION

LOW
01 02 03
04 05 06
07 08 09
10 11 12
HIGH

DINNER TIME: _____

FOOD & DRINK

INTENSITY/REACTION

LOW
01 02 03
04 05 06
07 08 09
10 11 12
HIGH

SYMPTOMS -

PAIN MEASUREMENT SCALE

0 1 2 3 4 5 6 7 8 9 10

No Pain | Mild | Moderate | Severe | Very Severe | Worst Pain Possible

WATER TRACKER

1 2 3 4
5 6 7 8

STRESS LEVEL

BRISTOL STOOL CHART

TYPE 1 – HARD LUMPS ☐
TYPE 2 – LUMPY ☐
TYPE 3 – CRACKED ☐
TYPE 4 – SMOOTH ☐
TYPE 5 – SOFT BLOBS ☐
TYPE 6 – MUSHY EDGES ☐
TYPE 7 – JUST LIQUID ☐

NOTES

Daily IBS Diary

Date: ....

BREAKFAST TIME: _____

LUNCH TIME: _____

DINNER TIME: _____

FOOD & DRINK

INTENSITY/REACTION

LOW
- 01 02 03
- 04 05 06
- 07 08 09
- 10 11 12 HIGH

FOOD & DRINK

INTENSITY/REACTION

LOW
- 01 02 03
- 04 05 06
- 07 08 09
- 10 11 12 HIGH

FOOD & DRINK

INTENSITY/REACTION

LOW
- 01 02 03
- 04 05 06
- 07 08 09
- 10 11 12 HIGH

SYMPTOMS -

PAIN MEASUREMENT SCALE

0 1 2 3 4 5 6 7 8 9 10

No Pain | Mild | Moderate | Severe | Very Severe | Worst Pain Possible

WATER TRACKER

1 2 3 4
5 6 7 8

STRESS LEVEL

BRISTOL STOOL CHART

- TYPE 1 – HARD LUMPS ☐
- TYPE 2 – LUMPY ☐
- TYPE 3 – CRACKED ☐
- TYPE 4 – SMOOTH ☐
- TYPE 5 – SOFT BLOBS ☐
- TYPE 6 – MUSHY EDGES ☐
- TYPE 7 – JUST LIQUID ☐

NOTES

Daily IBS Diary

Date: ....

BREAKFAST TIME: _____

LUNCH TIME: _____

DINNER TIME: _____

FOOD & DRINK

INTENSITY/REACTION

LOW 01 02 03
04 05 06
07 08 09
10 11 12 HIGH

FOOD & DRINK

INTENSITY/REACTION

LOW 01 02 03
04 05 06
07 08 09
10 11 12 HIGH

FOOD & DRINK

INTENSITY/REACTION

LOW 01 02 03
04 05 06
07 08 09
10 11 12 HIGH

SYMPTOMS -

PAIN MEASUREMENT SCALE

0 1 2 3 4 5 6 7 8 9 10

No Pain | Mild | Moderate | Severe | Very Severe | Worst Pain Possible

WATER TRACKER

1 2 3 4
5 6 7 8

STRESS LEVEL

BRISTOL STOOL CHART

TYPE 1 – HARD LUMPS ☐

TYPE 2 – LUMPY ☐

TYPE 3 – CRACKED ☐

TYPE 4 – SMOOTH ☐

TYPE 5 – SOFT BLOBS ☐

TYPE 6 – MUSHY EDGES ☐

TYPE 7 – JUST LIQUID ☐

NOTES

Daily IBS Diary

Date: ....

BREAKFAST TIME: _____

FOOD & DRINK

INTENSITY/REACTION

LOW 01 02 03 04 05 06 07 08 09 10 11 12 HIGH

LUNCH TIME: _____

FOOD & DRINK

INTENSITY/REACTION

LOW 01 02 03 04 05 06 07 08 09 10 11 12 HIGH

DINNER TIME: _____

FOOD & DRINK

INTENSITY/REACTION

LOW 01 02 03 04 05 06 07 08 09 10 11 12 HIGH

SYMPTOMS -

PAIN MEASUREMENT SCALE

0 1 2 3 4 5 6 7 8 9 10

No Pain — Mild — Moderate — Severe — Very Severe — Worst Pain Possible

WATER TRACKER
1 2 3 4
5 6 7 8

STRESS LEVEL

BRISTOL STOOL CHART

TYPE 1 – HARD LUMPS ☐

TYPE 2 – LUMPY ☐

TYPE 3 – CRACKED ☐

TYPE 4 – SMOOTH ☐

TYPE 5 – SOFT BLOBS ☐

TYPE 6 – MUSHY EDGES ☐

TYPE 7 – JUST LIQUID ☐

NOTES

Daily IBS Diary

Date: ....

BREAKFAST TIME: _____

FOOD & DRINK

INTENSITY/REACTION

LOW
01 02 03
04 05 06
07 08 09
10 11 12
HIGH

LUNCH TIME: _____

FOOD & DRINK

INTENSITY/REACTION

LOW
01 02 03
04 05 06
07 08 09
10 11 12
HIGH

DINNER TIME: _____

FOOD & DRINK

INTENSITY/REACTION

LOW
01 02 03
04 05 06
07 08 09
10 11 12
HIGH

SYMPTOMS -

PAIN MEASUREMENT SCALE

0 1 2 3 4 5 6 7 8 9 10

No Pain | Mild | Moderate | Severe | Very Severe | Worst Pain Possible

WATER TRACKER
1 2 3 4
5 6 7 8

STRESS LEVEL

BRISTOL STOOL CHART

TYPE 1 – HARD LUMPS ☐

TYPE 2 – LUMPY ☐

TYPE 3 – CRACKED ☐

TYPE 4 – SMOOTH ☐

TYPE 5 – SOFT BLOBS ☐

TYPE 6 – MUSHY EDGES ☐

TYPE 7 – JUST LIQUID ☐

NOTES

Daily IBS Diary

Date: ....

BREAKFAST TIME: _____

FOOD & DRINK

INTENSITY/REACTION

LOW 01 02 03
04 05 06
07 08 09
10 11 12 HIGH

LUNCH TIME: _____

FOOD & DRINK

INTENSITY/REACTION

LOW 01 02 03
04 05 06
07 08 09
10 11 12 HIGH

DINNER TIME: _____

FOOD & DRINK

INTENSITY/REACTION

LOW 01 02 03
04 05 06
07 08 09
10 11 12 HIGH

SYMPTOMS -

PAIN MEASUREMENT SCALE

0 1 2 3 4 5 6 7 8 9 10

No Pain | Mild | Moderate | Severe | Very Severe | Worst Pain Possible

WATER TRACKER

1 2 3 4
5 6 7 8

STRESS LEVEL

BRISTOL STOOL CHART

TYPE 1 – HARD LUMPS ☐
TYPE 2 – LUMPY ☐
TYPE 3 – CRACKED ☐
TYPE 4 – SMOOTH ☐
TYPE 5 – SOFT BLOBS ☐
TYPE 6 – MUSHY EDGES ☐
TYPE 7 – JUST LIQUID ☐

NOTES

Daily IBS Diary

Date: ....

BREAKFAST TIME: _____

FOOD & DRINK

INTENSITY/REACTION

LOW
01 02 03
04 05 06
07 08 09
10 11 12
HIGH

LUNCH TIME: _____

FOOD & DRINK

INTENSITY/REACTION

LOW
01 02 03
04 05 06
07 08 09
10 11 12
HIGH

DINNER TIME: _____

FOOD & DRINK

INTENSITY/REACTION

LOW
01 02 03
04 05 06
07 08 09
10 11 12
HIGH

SYMPTOMS -

PAIN MEASUREMENT SCALE

0 1 2 3 4 5 6 7 8 9 10

No Pain | Mild | Moderate | Severe | Very Severe | Worst Pain Possible

WATER TRACKER

1 2 3 4
5 6 7 8

STRESS LEVEL

BRISTOL STOOL CHART

TYPE 1 – HARD LUMPS ☐

TYPE 2 – LUMPY ☐

TYPE 3 – CRACKED ☐

TYPE 4 – SMOOTH ☐

TYPE 5 – SOFT BLOBS ☐

TYPE 6 – MUSHY EDGES ☐

TYPE 7 – JUST LIQUID ☐

NOTES

Daily IBS Diary

Date: ....

BREAKFAST TIME: _____

FOOD & DRINK

INTENSITY/REACTION

LOW
- 01 02 03
- 04 05 06
- 07 08 09
- 10 11 12
HIGH

LUNCH TIME: _____

FOOD & DRINK

INTENSITY/REACTION

LOW
- 01 02 03
- 04 05 06
- 07 08 09
- 10 11 12
HIGH

DINNER TIME: _____

FOOD & DRINK

INTENSITY/REACTION

LOW
- 01 02 03
- 04 05 06
- 07 08 09
- 10 11 12
HIGH

SYMPTOMS -

PAIN MEASUREMENT SCALE

0 1 2 3 4 5 6 7 8 9 10

No Pain | Mild | Moderate | Severe | Very Severe | Worst Pain Possible

WATER TRACKER

1 2 3 4
5 6 7 8

STRESS LEVEL

BRISTOL STOOL CHART

TYPE 1 – HARD LUMPS ☐

TYPE 2 – LUMPY ☐

TYPE 3 – CRACKED ☐

TYPE 4 – SMOOTH ☐

TYPE 5 – SOFT BLOBS ☐

TYPE 6 – MUSHY EDGES ☐

TYPE 7 – JUST LIQUID ☐

NOTES

Daily IBS Diary

Date: ....

BREAKFAST TIME: _____

FOOD & DRINK

INTENSITY/REACTION

LOW 01 02 03
04 05 06
07 08 09
10 11 12 HIGH

LUNCH TIME: _____

FOOD & DRINK

INTENSITY/REACTION

LOW 01 02 03
04 05 06
07 08 09
10 11 12 HIGH

DINNER TIME: _____

FOOD & DRINK

INTENSITY/REACTION

LOW 01 02 03
04 05 06
07 08 09
10 11 12 HIGH

SYMPTOMS -

PAIN MEASUREMENT SCALE

0 1 2 3 4 5 6 7 8 9 10

No Pain — Mild — Moderate — Severe — Very Severe — Worst Pain Possible

WATER TRACKER
1 2 3 4
5 6 7 8

STRESS LEVEL

BRISTOL STOOL CHART

TYPE 1 – HARD LUMPS ☐

TYPE 2 – LUMPY ☐

TYPE 3 – CRACKED ☐

TYPE 4 – SMOOTH ☐

TYPE 5 – SOFT BLOBS ☐

TYPE 6 – MUSHY EDGES ☐

TYPE 7 – JUST LIQUID ☐

NOTES

Daily IBS Diary

Date: ....

BREAKFAST TIME: _____

FOOD & DRINK

INTENSITY/REACTION
LOW
01 02 03
04 05 06
07 08 09
10 11 12 HIGH

LUNCH TIME: _____

FOOD & DRINK

INTENSITY/REACTION
LOW
01 02 03
04 05 06
07 08 09
10 11 12 HIGH

DINNER TIME: _____

FOOD & DRINK

INTENSITY/REACTION
LOW
01 02 03
04 05 06
07 08 09
10 11 12 HIGH

SYMPTOMS -

PAIN MEASUREMENT SCALE

0 1 2 3 4 5 6 7 8 9 10

No Pain | Mild | Moderate | Severe | Very Severe | Worst Pain Possible

WATER TRACKER
1 2 3 4
5 6 7 8

STRESS LEVEL

BRISTOL STOOL CHART

TYPE 1 – HARD LUMPS ☐

TYPE 2 – LUMPY ☐

TYPE 3 – CRACKED ☐

TYPE 4 – SMOOTH ☐

TYPE 5 – SOFT BLOBS ☐

TYPE 6 – MUSHY EDGES ☐

TYPE 7 – JUST LIQUID ☐

NOTES

Daily IBS Diary

Date: ....

BREAKFAST TIME: _____

FOOD & DRINK

INTENSITY/REACTION

LOW
01 02 03
04 05 06
07 08 09
10 11 12 HIGH

LUNCH TIME: _____

FOOD & DRINK

INTENSITY/REACTION

LOW
01 02 03
04 05 06
07 08 09
10 11 12 HIGH

DINNER TIME: _____

FOOD & DRINK

INTENSITY/REACTION

LOW
01 02 03
04 05 06
07 08 09
10 11 12 HIGH

SYMPTOMS -

PAIN MEASUREMENT SCALE

0 1 2 3 4 5 6 7 8 9 10

No Pain | Mild | Moderate | Severe | Very Severe | Worst Pain Possible

WATER TRACKER

1 2 3 4
5 6 7 8

STRESS LEVEL

BRISTOL STOOL CHART

TYPE 1 - HARD LUMPS ☐

TYPE 2 - LUMPY ☐

TYPE 3 - CRACKED ☐

TYPE 4 - SMOOTH ☐

TYPE 5 - SOFT BLOBS ☐

TYPE 6 - MUSHY EDGES ☐

TYPE 7 - JUST LIQUID ☐

NOTES

Daily IBS Diary

Date: ....

BREAKFAST TIME: _____

LUNCH TIME: _____

DINNER TIME: _____

FOOD & DRINK (Breakfast)

INTENSITY/REACTION
LOW 01 02 03
04 05 06
07 08 09
10 11 12 HIGH

FOOD & DRINK (Lunch)

INTENSITY/REACTION
LOW 01 02 03
04 05 06
07 08 09
10 11 12 HIGH

FOOD & DRINK (Dinner)

INTENSITY/REACTION
LOW 01 02 03
04 05 06
07 08 09
10 11 12 HIGH

SYMPTOMS -

PAIN MEASUREMENT SCALE

0 1 2 3 4 5 6 7 8 9 10

No Pain | Mild | Moderate | Severe | Very Severe | Worst Pain Possible

WATER TRACKER
1 2 3 4
5 6 7 8

STRESS LEVEL

BRISTOL STOOL CHART

TYPE 1 – HARD LUMPS ☐

TYPE 2 – LUMPY ☐

TYPE 3 – CRACKED ☐

TYPE 4 – SMOOTH ☐

TYPE 5 – SOFT BLOBS ☐

TYPE 6 – MUSHY EDGES ☐

TYPE 7 – JUST LIQUID ☐

NOTES

Daily IBS Diary

Date: ....

BREAKFAST TIME: _____

FOOD & DRINK

INTENSITY/REACTION

LOW
- 01
- 02
- 03
- 04
- 05
- 06
- 07
- 08
- 09
- 10
- 11
- 12
HIGH

LUNCH TIME: _____

FOOD & DRINK

INTENSITY/REACTION

LOW
- 01
- 02
- 03
- 04
- 05
- 06
- 07
- 08
- 09
- 10
- 11
- 12
HIGH

DINNER TIME: _____

FOOD & DRINK

INTENSITY/REACTION

LOW
- 01
- 02
- 03
- 04
- 05
- 06
- 07
- 08
- 09
- 10
- 11
- 12
HIGH

SYMPTOMS -

PAIN MEASUREMENT SCALE

0 1 2 3 4 5 6 7 8 9 10

- No Pain
- Mild
- Moderate
- Severe
- Very Severe
- Worst Pain Possible

WATER TRACKER

1 2 3 4
5 6 7 8

STRESS LEVEL

BRISTOL STOOL CHART

- TYPE 1 – HARD LUMPS ☐
- TYPE 2 – LUMPY ☐
- TYPE 3 – CRACKED ☐
- TYPE 4 – SMOOTH ☐
- TYPE 5 – SOFT BLOBS ☐
- TYPE 6 – MUSHY EDGES ☐
- TYPE 7 – JUST LIQUID ☐

NOTES

Daily IBS Diary

Date: ....

BREAKFAST TIME: _____

FOOD & DRINK

INTENSITY/REACTION

LOW
01 02 03
04 05 06
07 08 09
10 11 12 HIGH

LUNCH TIME: _____

FOOD & DRINK

INTENSITY/REACTION

LOW
01 02 03
04 05 06
07 08 09
10 11 12 HIGH

DINNER TIME: _____

FOOD & DRINK

INTENSITY/REACTION

LOW
01 02 03
04 05 06
07 08 09
10 11 12 HIGH

SYMPTOMS -

PAIN MEASUREMENT SCALE

0 1 2 3 4 5 6 7 8 9 10

No Pain | Mild | Moderate | Severe | Very Severe | Worst Pain Possible

WATER TRACKER

1 2 3 4
5 6 7 8

STRESS LEVEL

BRISTOL STOOL CHART

TYPE 1 – HARD LUMPS ☐

TYPE 2 – LUMPY ☐

TYPE 3 – CRACKED ☐

TYPE 4 – SMOOTH ☐

TYPE 5 – SOFT BLOBS ☐

TYPE 6 – MUSHY EDGES ☐

TYPE 7 – JUST LIQUID ☐

NOTES

Daily IBS Diary

Date: ....

BREAKFAST TIME: _____

FOOD & DRINK

INTENSITY/REACTION

LOW 01 02 03
04 05 06
07 08 09
10 11 12 HIGH

LUNCH TIME: _____

FOOD & DRINK

INTENSITY/REACTION

LOW 01 02 03
04 05 06
07 08 09
10 11 12 HIGH

DINNER TIME: _____

FOOD & DRINK

INTENSITY/REACTION

LOW 01 02 03
04 05 06
07 08 09
10 11 12 HIGH

SYMPTOMS -

PAIN MEASUREMENT SCALE

0 1 2 3 4 5 6 7 8 9 10

No Pain | Mild | Moderate | Severe | Very Severe | Worst Pain Possible

WATER TRACKER

1 2 3 4
5 6 7 8

STRESS LEVEL

BRISTOL STOOL CHART

TYPE 1 – HARD LUMPS ☐

TYPE 2 – LUMPY ☐

TYPE 3 – CRACKED ☐

TYPE 4 – SMOOTH ☐

TYPE 5 – SOFT BLOBS ☐

TYPE 6 – MUSHY EDGES ☐

TYPE 7 – JUST LIQUID ☐

NOTES

Daily IBS Diary

Date: ....

BREAKFAST TIME: _____

FOOD & DRINK

INTENSITY/REACTION

LOW 01 02 03
04 05 06
07 08 09
10 11 12 HIGH

LUNCH TIME: _____

FOOD & DRINK

INTENSITY/REACTION

LOW 01 02 03
04 05 06
07 08 09
10 11 12 HIGH

DINNER TIME: _____

FOOD & DRINK

INTENSITY/REACTION

LOW 01 02 03
04 05 06
07 08 09
10 11 12 HIGH

SYMPTOMS -

PAIN MEASUREMENT SCALE

0 1 2 3 4 5 6 7 8 9 10

No Pain | Mild | Moderate | Severe | Very Severe | Worst Pain Possible

WATER TRACKER

1 2 3 4
5 6 7 8

STRESS LEVEL

BRISTOL STOOL CHART

TYPE 1 – HARD LUMPS ☐
TYPE 2 – LUMPY ☐
TYPE 3 – CRACKED ☐
TYPE 4 – SMOOTH ☐
TYPE 5 – SOFT BLOBS ☐
TYPE 6 – MUSHY EDGES ☐
TYPE 7 – JUST LIQUID ☐

NOTES

Daily IBS Diary

Date: ....

BREAKFAST TIME: _____

FOOD & DRINK

INTENSITY/REACTION

LOW
01 02 03
04 05 06
07 08 09
10 11 12
HIGH

LUNCH TIME: _____

FOOD & DRINK

INTENSITY/REACTION

LOW
01 02 03
04 05 06
07 08 09
10 11 12
HIGH

DINNER TIME: _____

FOOD & DRINK

INTENSITY/REACTION

LOW
01 02 03
04 05 06
07 08 09
10 11 12
HIGH

SYMPTOMS -

PAIN MEASUREMENT SCALE

0 1 2 3 4 5 6 7 8 9 10

No Pain | Mild | Moderate | Severe | Very Severe | Worst Pain Possible

WATER TRACKER

1 2 3 4
5 6 7 8

STRESS LEVEL

BRISTOL STOOL CHART

TYPE 1 – HARD LUMPS ☐

TYPE 2 – LUMPY ☐

TYPE 3 – CRACKED ☐

TYPE 4 – SMOOTH ☐

TYPE 5 – SOFT BLOBS ☐

TYPE 6 – MUSHY EDGES ☐

TYPE 7 – JUST LIQUID ☐

NOTES

Daily IBS Diary

Date: ....

BREAKFAST TIME: _____

FOOD & DRINK

INTENSITY/REACTION

LOW
01 02 03
04 05 06
07 08 09
10 11 12
HIGH

LUNCH TIME: _____

FOOD & DRINK

INTENSITY/REACTION

LOW
01 02 03
04 05 06
07 08 09
10 11 12
HIGH

DINNER TIME: _____

FOOD & DRINK

INTENSITY/REACTION

LOW
01 02 03
04 05 06
07 08 09
10 11 12
HIGH

SYMPTOMS -

PAIN MEASUREMENT SCALE

0 1 2 3 4 5 6 7 8 9 10

No Pain | Mild | Moderate | Severe | Very Severe | Worst Pain Possible

WATER TRACKER

1 2 3 4
5 6 7 8

STRESS LEVEL

BRISTOL STOOL CHART

TYPE 1 – HARD LUMPS ☐

TYPE 2 – LUMPY ☐

TYPE 3 – CRACKED ☐

TYPE 4 – SMOOTH ☐

TYPE 5 – SOFT BLOBS ☐

TYPE 6 – MUSHY EDGES ☐

TYPE 7 – JUST LIQUID ☐

NOTES

Daily IBS Diary

Date: ....

BREAKFAST TIME: _____

LUNCH TIME: _____

DINNER TIME: _____

FOOD & DRINK

INTENSITY/REACTION

LOW 01 02 03
     04 05 06
     07 08 09
     10 11 12 HIGH

FOOD & DRINK

INTENSITY/REACTION

LOW 01 02 03
     04 05 06
     07 08 09
     10 11 12 HIGH

FOOD & DRINK

INTENSITY/REACTION

LOW 01 02 03
     04 05 06
     07 08 09
     10 11 12 HIGH

SYMPTOMS -

PAIN MEASUREMENT SCALE

0 1 2 3 4 5 6 7 8 9 10

No Pain | Mild | Moderate | Severe | Very Severe | Worst Pain Possible

WATER TRACKER

1 2 3 4
5 6 7 8

STRESS LEVEL

BRISTOL STOOL CHART

TYPE 1 – HARD LUMPS ☐

TYPE 2 – LUMPY ☐

TYPE 3 – CRACKED ☐

TYPE 4 – SMOOTH ☐

TYPE 5 – SOFT BLOBS ☐

TYPE 6 – MUSHY EDGES ☐

TYPE 7 – JUST LIQUID ☐

NOTES

Daily IBS Diary

Date: ....

BREAKFAST TIME: _____

FOOD & DRINK

INTENSITY/REACTION

LOW
- 01 02 03
- 04 05 06
- 07 08 09
- 10 11 12 HIGH

LUNCH TIME: _____

FOOD & DRINK

INTENSITY/REACTION

LOW
- 01 02 03
- 04 05 06
- 07 08 09
- 10 11 12 HIGH

DINNER TIME: _____

FOOD & DRINK

INTENSITY/REACTION

LOW
- 01 02 03
- 04 05 06
- 07 08 09
- 10 11 12 HIGH

SYMPTOMS -

PAIN MEASUREMENT SCALE

0 1 2 3 4 5 6 7 8 9 10

No Pain | Mild | Moderate | Severe | Very Severe | Worst Pain Possible

WATER TRACKER
1 2 3 4
5 6 7 8

STRESS LEVEL

BRISTOL STOOL CHART

TYPE 1 – HARD LUMPS ☐

TYPE 2 – LUMPY ☐

TYPE 3 – CRACKED ☐

TYPE 4 – SMOOTH ☐

TYPE 5 – SOFT BLOBS ☐

TYPE 6 – MUSHY EDGES ☐

TYPE 7 – JUST LIQUID ☐

NOTES

Daily IBS Diary

Date: ....

BREAKFAST TIME: _____

LUNCH TIME: _____

DINNER TIME: _____

FOOD & DRINK

INTENSITY/REACTION

LOW
01 02 03
04 05 06
07 08 09
10 11 12
HIGH

FOOD & DRINK

INTENSITY/REACTION

LOW
01 02 03
04 05 06
07 08 09
10 11 12
HIGH

FOOD & DRINK

INTENSITY/REACTION

LOW
01 02 03
04 05 06
07 08 09
10 11 12
HIGH

SYMPTOMS -

PAIN MEASUREMENT SCALE

0 1 2 3 4 5 6 7 8 9 10

No Pain | Mild | Moderate | Severe | Very Severe | Worst Pain Possible

WATER TRACKER

1 2 3 4
5 6 7 8

STRESS LEVEL

BRISTOL STOOL CHART

TYPE 1 – HARD LUMPS ☐

TYPE 2 – LUMPY ☐

TYPE 3 – CRACKED ☐

TYPE 4 – SMOOTH ☐

TYPE 5 – SOFT BLOBS ☐

TYPE 6 – MUSHY EDGES ☐

TYPE 7 – JUST LIQUID ☐

NOTES

Daily IBS Diary

Date: ....

BREAKFAST TIME: _____

FOOD & DRINK

INTENSITY/REACTION

LOW 01 02 03
     04 05 06
     07 08 09
     10 11 12 HIGH

LUNCH TIME: _____

FOOD & DRINK

INTENSITY/REACTION

LOW 01 02 03
     04 05 06
     07 08 09
     10 11 12 HIGH

DINNER TIME: _____

FOOD & DRINK

INTENSITY/REACTION

LOW 01 02 03
     04 05 06
     07 08 09
     10 11 12 HIGH

SYMPTOMS -

PAIN MEASUREMENT SCALE

0 1 2 3 4 5 6 7 8 9 10

No Pain | Mild | Moderate | Severe | Very Severe | Worst Pain Possible

WATER TRACKER

1 2 3 4
5 6 7 8

STRESS LEVEL

BRISTOL STOOL CHART

TYPE 1 – HARD LUMPS ☐
TYPE 2 – LUMPY ☐
TYPE 3 – CRACKED ☐
TYPE 4 – SMOOTH ☐
TYPE 5 – SOFT BLOBS ☐
TYPE 6 – MUSHY EDGES ☐
TYPE 7 – JUST LIQUID ☐

NOTES

Monthly
BOWEL MOVEMENT TRACKER

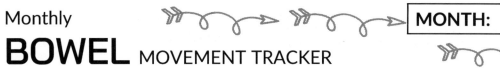

MONTH:

	MOVEMENT		Description of stool condition and color		Number of times I passed stools today				Treatment / Bowel Aids
	YES	NO	Regular	Constipation					
1									
2									
3									
4									
5									
6									
7									
8									
9									
10									
11									
12									
13									
14									
15									
16									
17									
18									
19									
20									
21									
22									
23									
24									
25									
26									
27									
28									
29									
30									
31									

Monthly BOWEL MOVEMENT TRACKER

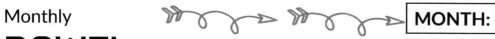

MONTH:

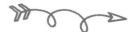

#	MOVEMENT - YES	MOVEMENT - NO	Description of stool condition and color - Regular	Description of stool condition and color - Constipation	Number of times I passed stools today			Treatment / Bowel Aids
1								
2								
3								
4								
5								
6								
7								
8								
9								
10								
11								
12								
13								
14								
15								
16								
17								
18								
19								
20								
21								
22								
23								
24								
25								
26								
27								
28								
29								
30								
31								

Monthly BOWEL MOVEMENT TRACKER

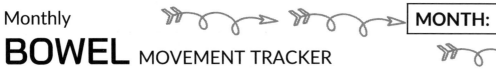

MONTH:

#	MOVEMENT YES	MOVEMENT NO	Description of stool condition and color — Regular	Description of stool condition and color — Constipation	Number of times I passed stools today				Treatment / Bowel Aids
1									
2									
3									
4									
5									
6									
7									
8									
9									
10									
11									
12									
13									
14									
15									
16									
17									
18									
19									
20									
21									
22									
23									
24									
25									
26									
27									
28									
29									
30									
31									

Abnormal BOWEL MOVEMENT TRACKER

MONTH:

Date	Time	Type*	Description and Color of Abnormal Stools	Possible Cause	Treatment

*TYPES: 1, 2, 3, 4, 5, 6, 7 based on Bristol Stool Chart definitions

NOTES

Abnormal BOWEL MOVEMENT TRACKER

MONTH:

Date	Time	Type*	Description and Color of Abnormal Stools	Possible Cause	Treatment

*TYPES: 1, 2, 3, 4, 5, 6, 7 based on Bristol Stool Chart definitions

NOTES

Abnormal BOWEL MOVEMENT TRACKER

MONTH:

Date	Time	Type*	Description and Color of Abnormal Stools	Possible Cause	Treatment

*TYPES: 1, 2, 3, 4, 5, 6, 7 based on Bristol Stool Chart definitions

NOTES

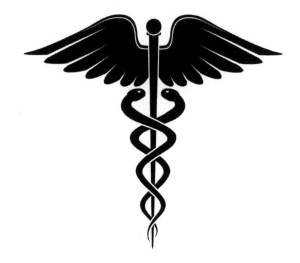

SECTION 2

APPOINTMENTS & RECORDS

MEDICAL APPOINTMENTS

Date	Time	Doctor	Contact
Reason for Visit		**Questions**	**Outcome**
			Medication Prescribed
Notes			**Treatment**
			Follow up

Date	Time	Doctor	Contact
Reason for Visit		**Questions**	**Outcome**
			Medication Prescribed
Notes			**Treatment**
			Follow up

Date	Time	Doctor	Contact
Reason for Visit		**Questions**	**Outcome**
			Medication Prescribed
Notes			**Treatment**
			Follow up

MEDICAL APPOINTMENTS

Date	Time	Doctor	Contact
Reason for Visit		Questions	Outcome
			Medication Prescribed
Notes			Treatment
			Follow up

Date	Time	Doctor	Contact
Reason for Visit		Questions	Outcome
			Medication Prescribed
Notes			**Treatment**
			Follow up

Date	Time	Doctor	Contact
Reason for Visit		Questions	Outcome
			Medication Prescribed
Notes			**Treatment**
			Follow up

MEDICAL APPOINTMENTS

Date	Time	Doctor	Contact
Reason for Visit		Questions	Outcome
			Medication Prescribed
Notes			Treatment
			Follow up

Date	Time	Doctor	Contact
Reason for Visit		**Questions**	**Outcome**
			Medication Prescribed
Notes			**Treatment**
			Follow up

Date	Time	Doctor	Contact
Reason for Visit		**Questions**	**Outcome**
			Medication Prescribed
Notes			**Treatment**
			Follow up

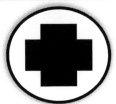

SYMPTOMS RECORD

DATE		Food, Medication or Activity:	Symptoms:	MILD	MODERATE	SEVERE
TIME						
NOTES						

DATE		Food, Medication or Activity:	Symptoms:	MILD	MODERATE	SEVERE
TIME						
NOTES						

DATE		Food, Medication or Activity:	Symptoms:	MILD	MODERATE	SEVERE
TIME						
NOTES						

DATE		Food, Medication or Activity:	Symptoms:	MILD	MODERATE	SEVERE
TIME						
NOTES						

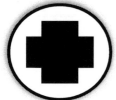

SYMPTOMS RECORD

DATE		Food, Medication or Activity:	Symptoms:	MILD	MODERATE	SEVERE
TIME						
NOTES						

DATE		Food, Medication or Activity:	Symptoms:	MILD	MODERATE	SEVERE
TIME						
NOTES						

DATE		Food, Medication or Activity:	Symptoms:	MILD	MODERATE	SEVERE
TIME						
NOTES						

DATE		Food, Medication or Activity:	Symptoms:	MILD	MODERATE	SEVERE
TIME						
NOTES						

MEDICATION RECORD

Doctor		Tel	
Pharmacy		Tel	

Start Date	End Date	Medication	Dosage	Breakfast	Lunch	Dinner	Other Times	Notes

MEDICATION RECORD

Doctor		Tel	
Pharmacy		Tel	

Start Date	End Date	Medication	Dosage	Breakfast	Lunch	Dinner	Other Times	Notes

WEEKLY MEDICATION RECORD

For		
Doctor		Tel
WEEK OF		

Medication	Dosage	Time(s)	M	T	W	T	F	S	S

Notes / Side Effects

WEEKLY MEDICATION RECORD

For			
Doctor		Tel	
WEEK OF			

Medication	Dosage	Time(s)	M	T	W	T	F	S	S

Notes / Side Effects

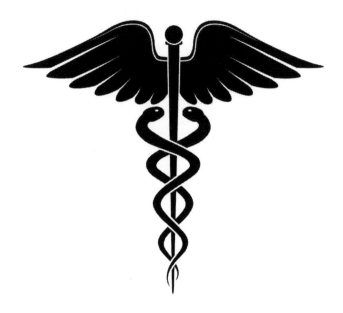

SECTION 3

LOW FODMAP ALLOWED FOODS, MEAL PLANNERS & SHOPPING LISTS

So, What Exactly are FODMAPs?

Basically, FODMAPs are short chain carbohydrates and sugar alcohols that the body often has difficulty digesting. Consequently, they can ferment in your large intestine (bowel) during digestion, and then several processes take place that causes the intestine to resulting in symptoms such as pain and bloating that are commonly recognized in disorders such as IBS.

FODMAPs can be found naturally in some foods or they can be added such as the fructose in fruits and vegetables.

Whilst Fodmaps don't necessarily make the foods unhealthy for you and in many cases contain healthy prebiotics that assist in stimulating the growth of those beneficial bacteria you need. There are others that cause gastrointestinal symptoms for certain people when they are eating or drinking.

Does Following a low FODMAP diet help with IBS?

- Low FODMAP diets are frequently recommended to help many different types of digestive problems which include IBS.

- Low Fodmap diets are often suggested to assist with Small intestinal bacterial overgrowth (SIBO)

Some of the symptoms or signs that suggest you may be eating to many high FODMAP foods are:
- Gas
- Pain
- Bloating
- Abdominal pain
- Diarrhea
- Feeling overfull after eating or drinking only a small amount of food or liquid

A low FODMAPs diet may help relieve these problems, particularly in people with IBS.

ALLOWED FODMAP FOODS

Vegetables
Alfalfa sprouts
Bean sprouts
Bell pepper
Carrot
Green beans
Bok choy
Cucumber
Lettuce
Tomato
Zucchini
Bamboo shoots
Eggplant
Ginger
Chives
Olives
Parsnips
Potatoes
Turnips

Fresh Fruits
Oranges
Grapes
Honeydew melon
Cantaloupe
Banana
Blueberries
Grapefruit
Kiwi
Lemon
Lime
Oranges
Strawberries

Drinks
Tea and coffee (use non-dairy milk or creamers)
Fruit juice not from concentrate
Water

Dairy that is lactose-free, and hard cheeses, or ripened/matured cheeses including (If you are not lactose intolerant, you may not need to avoid dairy with lactose.)
Brie
Camembert
Feta cheese
Beef, pork, chicken, fish, eggs
Avoid breadcrumbs, marinades, and sauces/gravies that may be high in FODMAPs.
Soy products including tofu, tempeh

Grains
Rice
Rice bran
Oats
Oat bran
Quinoa
Corn flour
Sourdough spelt bread
Gluten-free bread and pasta
Gluten is not a FODMAP, but many gluten-free products tend to be low in FODMAPs.

Non-dairy milks
Almond milk
Rice milk
Coconut milk

Nuts and seeds
Almonds
Macadamia
Peanuts
Pine nuts
Walnuts (fewer than 10-15/serving for nuts)

FODMAPs TO AVOID

Some Vegetables
Onions
Garlic
Cabbage
Broccoli
Cauliflower
Snow peas
Asparagus
Artichokes
Leeks
Beetroot
Celery
Sweet corn
Brussels sprouts
Mushrooms

Fruits, particularly "stone" fruits like:
Peaches
Apricots
Nectarines
Plums
Prunes
Mangoes
Apples
Pears
Watermelon
Cherries
Blackberries
Dried fruits and fruit juice concentrate

Beans and Lentils

Wheat and Rye
Breads
Cereals
Pastas
Crackers
Pizza

Dairy products that contain lactose
Milk
Soft cheese
Yogurt
Ice cream
Custard
Pudding
Cottage cheese

Nuts, including cashews and pistachios

Sweeteners and artificial sweeteners
High fructose corn syrup
Honey
Agave nectar
Sorbitol
Xylitol
Maltitol
Mannitol
Isomalt (commonly found in sugar-free gum and mints, and even cough syrups)

Drinks
Alcohol
Sports drinks
Coconut water

Low FODMAP SHOPPING LIST

Meat, Fish & Poultry

Fruit & Vegetables

Condiments & Spreads

Drinks

Dairy

Cereals, Grains & Bakery

Cooking Ingredients

Low FODMAP SHOPPING LIST

Meat, Fish & Poultry

Fruit & Vegetables

Condiments & Spreads

Drinks

Dairy

Cereals, Grains & Bakery

Cooking Ingredients

Low FODMAP SHOPPING LIST

Meat, Fish & Poultry

Fruit & Vegetables

Condiments & Spreads

Dairy

Cereals, Grains & Bakery

Drinks

Cooking Ingredients

Low FODMAP SHOPPING LIST

Meat, Fish & Poultry

Fruit & Vegetables

Condiments & Spreads

Drinks

Dairy

Cereals, Grains & Bakery

Cooking Ingredients

Low FODMAP SHOPPING LIST

Meat, Fish & Poultry

Fruit & Vegetables

Condiments & Spreads

Drinks

Dairy

Cereals, Grains & Bakery

Cooking Ingredients

Low FODMAP SHOPPING LIST

Meat, Fish & Poultry

Fruit & Vegetables

Condiments & Spreads

Dairy

Cereals, Grains & Bakery

Drinks

Cooking Ingredients

Low FODMAP SHOPPING LIST

Meat, Fish & Poultry

Fruit & Vegetables

Condiments & Spreads

Dairy

Cereals, Grains & Bakery

Drinks

Cooking Ingredients

Low FODMAP SHOPPING LIST

Meat, Fish & Poultry

Fruit & Vegetables

Condiments & Spreads

Dairy

Cereals, Grains & Bakery

Drinks

Cooking Ingredients

Low FODMAP SHOPPING LIST

Meat, Fish & Poultry

Fruit & Vegetables

Condiments & Spreads

Dairy

Cereals, Grains & Bakery

Drinks

Cooking Ingredients

Low FODMAP SHOPPING LIST

Meat, Fish & Poultry

Fruit & Vegetables

Condiments & Spreads

Drinks

Dairy

Cereals, Grains & Bakery

Cooking Ingredients

Low FODMAP SHOPPING LIST

Meat, Fish & Poultry

Fruit & Vegetables

Condiments & Spreads

Drinks

Dairy

Cereals, Grains & Bakery

Cooking Ingredients

Low FODMAP SHOPPING LIST

Meat, Fish & Poultry

Fruit & Vegetables

Condiments & Spreads

Drinks

Dairy

Cereals, Grains & Bakery

Cooking Ingredients

FODMAP Meal Planner

	BREAKFAST	LUNCH	DINNER
MON			
TUES			
WED			
THU			
FRI			
SAT			
SUN			

FODMAP Meal Planner

	BREAKFAST	LUNCH	DINNER
MON			
TUES			
WED			
THU			
FRI			
SAT			
SUN			

FODMAP Meal Planner

	BREAKFAST	LUNCH	DINNER
MON			
TUES			
WED			
THU			
FRI			
SAT			
SUN			

FODMAP Meal Planner

	BREAKFAST	LUNCH	DINNER
MON			
TUES			
WED			
THU			
FRI			
SAT			
SUN			

FODMAP Meal Planner

	BREAKFAST	LUNCH	DINNER
MON			
TUES			
WED			
THU			
FRI			
SAT			
SUN			

FODMAP Meal Planner

	BREAKFAST	LUNCH	DINNER
MON			
TUES			
WED			
THU			
FRI			
SAT			
SUN			

FODMAP Meal Planner

	BREAKFAST	LUNCH	DINNER
MON			
TUES			
WED			
THU			
FRI			
SAT			
SUN			

FODMAP Meal Planner

	BREAKFAST	LUNCH	DINNER
MON			
TUES			
WED			
THU			
FRI			
SAT			
SUN			

FODMAP Meal Planner

	BREAKFAST	LUNCH	DINNER
MON			
TUES			
WED			
THU			
FRI			
SAT			
SUN			

FODMAP Meal Planner

	BREAKFAST	LUNCH	DINNER
MON			
TUES			
WED			
THU			
FRI			
SAT			
SUN			

FODMAP Meal Planner

	BREAKFAST	LUNCH	DINNER
MON			
TUES			
WED			
THU			
FRI			
SAT			
SUN			

FODMAP Meal Planner

	BREAKFAST	LUNCH	DINNER
MON			
TUES			
WED			
THU			
FRI			
SAT			
SUN			

Your FODMAP Food List

ALLOWED	NOT ALLOWED

Your FODMAP Food List

ALLOWED	NOT ALLOWED